Staying Healthy

Mike and Tricia Whiteside

CASSELL

Cassell Publishers Limited
Artillery House, Artillery Row
London SW1P 1RT

British Library Cataloguing in Publication Data

Whiteside, Mike
  Staying healthy
  1. Man. Health. Self-care
  I. Title II. Whiteside, Tricia
  613

ISBN 0-304-31666-0

Typeset by Litho Link Ltd., Welshpool, Powys, Wales.
Printed and bound in Great Britain by
Courier International Ltd, Tiptree, Essex

Staying
Healthy

Cassell Lifeguides

Cassell 'Lifeguides' are books for today's way of life. The increasing trend towards a 'self-help society' is an indication of the need for reliable, helpful information in book form, as less and less advice is offered elsewhere.

With this series, Cassell furthers its reputation as a publisher of useful, practical self-help books, and tackles subjects which are very much in line with today's lifestyles and problems. As people become increasingly aware that situations need to be looked at from all sides, they can turn to these books for realistic advice and encouragement.

Contents

Preface

This book is designed to help you consider your present day-to-day habits and the effect they have upon your general health. We hope to make you aware of the pitfalls which hinder healthy living. We also want to help you to become aware of your options and to accept responsibility for your choices in life.

Each of the chapters contains guidelines to help you adopt healthier habits. Our aim has been to present an approach to healthy living in terms which do not require previous medical knowledge. There are many more detailed and complicated books on each of the subjects we deal with, but this book will give you a good start.

It is our earnest wish that the information in our book will enable you to live a happier, healthier and more fulfilled life.

Mike and Tricia Whiteside
December 1988

Introduction

Good health rarely happens by chance. Some are lucky enough to be born with the sort of constitution which appears to take abuse in all quarters without failing (we all know the person with the lively 90-year-old grandad who survived the Somme, smokes 60 cigarettes a day and drinks like a fish!). However, the majority of us are not quite so robust and, unless we take care of ourselves, are prone to debilitating diseases. Recent times have shown a movement towards greater awareness of how our bodies work and of ways to achieve and maintain better health.

Over the past 100 years there has been a gradual shift in the types of diseases which are responsible for the majority of deaths. Infectious illness such as polio, tuberculosis, dysentery and diphtheria used to claim an alarming number of lives. Childbirth was very risky; mothers often died from puerperal fever, a postnatal infection arising from unsanitary conditions and midwives' ignorance of the hazards. Similarly, ignorance of the action of bacteria and the need for hygiene made most surgical operations highly dangerous.

On the other hand, one recent preventive measure which has saved thousands of lives is the passing of the compulsory seat belt laws. Throughout the sixties we were urged to 'belt-up', during the seventies we were implored to 'clunk-click every trip', but it still took an Act of Parliament to push the majority of us into actually wearing our seat belts on every car journey. That one, small, automatic action we perform each time we sit in the car is likely to save us from being thrown through the windscreen if unfortunate enough to be involved in a collision.

Even with all the evidence in favour of opting for

preventive, diagnostic medicine, the British National Health Service is deeply entrenched in the curative method: to heal rather than to hinder sickness. (Perhaps it should be renamed the National Sickness Service.) How different from the acupuncturists in China who are paid only whilst their patients are well! Think then how important it is for each of us to consider how preventing sickness is better than remedies. Every day we can put on our 'seat belts' for life by adopting a way of living which values the uniqueness of every individual.

Life is a 'terminal' condition, but while it goes on we have some options as to how to live it. Recognising these options is half the battle. We have the choice as to whether or not we take responsibility for our own health or leave it to someone else (usually the doctor) to pick up the pieces. In reading this book you have taken the decision (whether consciously or unconsciously) to begin learning about better health, and you can choose which information is relevant to you and to your lifestyle. We have not set out to provide 'cures' for a number of diseases, but to suggest ways of promoting self-help to better all-round health and so possibly preventing serious illness later.

We have written this book in the belief that each person is a whole make-up of physical, emotional, mental and spiritual parts which interact to form a unique being. Perhaps you have noticed that when you have an emotional upset in your life you are less resistant to germs and often become ill. For instance, cold germs are always present in your system, but for the most part do not cause you any problem. A certain set of conditions must prevail for you actually to catch a cold, such as a lowering of the body temperature, a particular vitamin deficiency, and possibly general fatigue or upset. However, because each of us is different, one person will have a mild chill whereas another might suffer a bad attack of flu, both caused by the same germ. When we become sick, our bodies may be trying to relay a message to us about ourselves and the way in which we live. It is necessary to listen to these messages and heed their warnings.

As children we often know instinctively what is good and

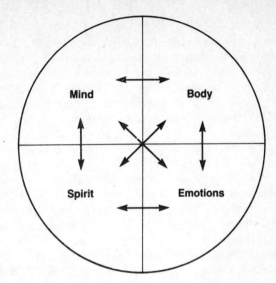

Interaction of mind, body, spirit and emotions

what is bad for us. Watch the beautiful posture of a 2-year-old: straight-spined and upright. A baby will often refuse food to which it is allergic. Unfortunately, as we mature and are subjected to the pressures of modern life, these instincts lose their force unless we make the conscious effort to be more aware of them. Many pregnant women find that they are more attuned than usual to their body's needs, and will crave foods which give them the nutrients their body requires or refuse those which may harm them. During the first few weeks of pregnancy the sense of taste changes, and often the first flavours which become abhorrent are those of alcohol and coffee, both of which contain stimulants which can be harmful to the body.

Western culture accepts that when a certain part of the body fails to function, it is best treated by the appropriate drug or surgical procedure in order to effect a 'cure'. Huge amounts of money are spent in seeking these 'cures' and training medical staff to use them. There exists a massive, international, multimillion pound drug industry which is continually pressurising doctors into prescribing their drugs. The 'miracles' promised to us from these procedures have lent credence to the myth that the medical profession is imbued with 'deity status', with control over life and death. There follows a certain amount of collusion between doctors and their patients, in that many people are quite happy to allow the physicians to take all the responsibility for the state of their health.

But it is now becoming obvious to many people that there is a price to pay for taking even small amounts of prescribed drugs which can have myriad side-effects and may, in themselves, lower the body's own defences to further infection. Indeed, present medical practice is so drug-orientated that patients may be ill from the mixtures of tablets they are consuming! This is not to say that we would condemn all drugs out of hand; there are some cases in which we consider them to be of vital importance. That said, however, this book concentrates on avoiding the necessity for medicines by encouraging basic healthy habits.

The mental attitude you have towards yourself and the way in which you treat your body is supremely important to your state of health. To lavish the right kind of care upon yourself gives your body the message to be fit and strong. If encouraged in this way, the body will draw on its own defence and immune systems in order to combat disease. Negative thoughts may cause damage to the system. For example, under great stress, large amounts of acid are released into the body, creating problems for the vital organs which require an acid/alkaline balance to function normally.

You can feel fitter and healthier by a gradual process that includes attention to diet (by eating the correct amounts of the right foods), proper exercise and breathing, adopting a healthy sleep pattern and, when necessary, knowing how to relax fully. The process should take your individual lifestyle into account. You have already taken the first step by choosing to read this book. Read on!

1
Lifestyles

It is possible thoughout life to go from day to day feeling 'under par' and yet not aware of it. Many people are generally unwell without being seriously ill; they 'exist' rather than live life to the full.

It would, of course, defeat the whole exercise if one allowed oneself to become over-anxious about the state of one's health! The accusation most frequently levelled at health writers is that 'You can't eat, drink or *do* anything without being told it will kill you!' This needs to be put into perspective. For instance, the effects over a number of years of large amounts of alcohol will eventually prove fatal. However, taken in small doses, alcohol may enhance your health. There is some evidence that red wine in particular helps to lower blood fats, which in turn keeps the arteries free of atheroma, the substance which clogs up the blood vessels causing heart attacks, strokes and thrombosis. Moderation is the key.

This chapter aims to help you identify the areas in your own life where improvements can be made to help you achieve a balanced way of life by expending your energies evenly in areas of work, leisure pursuits and relaxation. It also puts forward some ideas on factors which might have an adverse effect on your health.

The inheritance factor

The genes which you have inherited from parents and previous forebears will have some bearing on your health. If there is a family history of heart disease, cancer, allergies, rheumatism, mental disorders, etc., this will increase the chances of your being affected by the same disease. However, this does not mean that it is inevitable. If you are aware that you may be prone to a certain illness, it might be possible to take steps to avoid it. For example, if you have a family history of heart disease it is important not to become overweight, not to have a diet loaded with saturated fats, and to take a reasonable amount of exercise in order to minimise the risks.

You could draw your own family history chart putting in all the details you know to see if any disease is prevalent in your own family. You can make your chart as detailed as you wish. If one particular illness is present in both sides of the family, then this obviously increases your risk of contracting it.

Personal development

Personality type is something with which we are born and it affects the way in which we react to any given situation. However, from day one of life individuals are influenced by circumstances and by the people with whom they have close contact.

The scope for personal growth is infinite, but because none of us is perfect or living in a perfect world there are areas in our own personal development which may be damaged or stunted, and this is reflected in our behaviour. Throughout life we collect 'emotional luggage' and often become weighed down by it. When given a chance, the mind will naturally seek to heal the emotional wounds incurred by past hurts, sorting out the 'excess baggage' by consolidating and off-loading where appropriate. Life events such as a birth, death or other major happening may stir painful memories long since given over to the unconscious, confronting us with certain feelings about ourselves which give rise to anger or fear. Should these painful feelings be denied rather than faced, depression will usually result.

We are continually presented with opportunities for understanding and self-knowledge which will allow subsequent

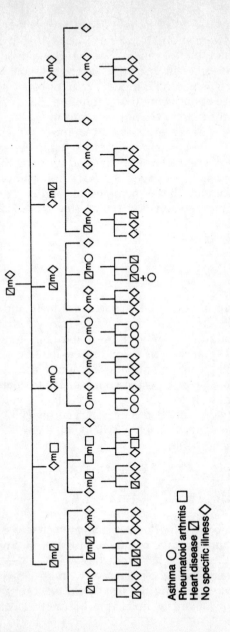

Lifestyles · 7

A family history diagram. This shows four generations of a family and
how three specific diseases might be passed down. It illustrates especially
how the chances of suffering from these diseases are greatly increased
should both parents have the same illness.

Asthma ○
Rheumatoid arthritis □
Heart disease ▨
No specific illness ◇

healing to take place. This process of maturing gives insight into the self, which in turn improves relationships both with ourselves and with others. Self-hate is one of the most destructive forces in existence. Do not discount how important your state of mind is in the search for better health, or allow prejudice about being thought of as a 'head case' to interfere with your search. Do not be afraid to ask for help.

There are now a large number of therapists working in different ways who aim to help people locked into destructive and painful behaviour patterns to come to terms with their emotional hang-ups (see page 29). It is important when contemplating any of these therapies to find a therapist who suits your own personality type, as the methods used vary enormously.

Attitude

The attitude which you hold towards yourself and your health will greatly determine your welfare. It may be that you have gone through life without even thinking how you regard illness. Do you see it as a sign of weakness or perhaps as a way of gaining care and attention? Your attitude will be apparent in almost every aspect of your life. Try to determine also your own attitude to your body, as it will give you good clues as to how you feel about yourself. Learning to have a loving attitude towards yourself will help you enormously in your quest for good health.

Body and soul?

'So, what's it all about, Alfie?' is a question which few mortals past the age of puberty have not asked of life itself. Spiritual health is something which has tended to be left to the clergy of multifarious religions, who often seek to impose their own beliefs on others. Following the last world war, religion as such has become distinctly unfashionable in this country, although there has been a very recent trend towards interest in all matters spiritual.

The perplexing nature of 'life force' has not been made any less confusing by the development of medical technology. In fact, there has been a large-scale crisis within the medical profession over what constitutes a death and when it should be pronounced. A body can be kept warm and breathing for an indefinite period even if 'brain death' has occurred. Very little, apart from the physical, is understood about coma. Do we, perhaps, leave people in a limbo of being neither dead nor alive? It would seem that the piece of puzzle which is missing from this picture is that of the spirit.

It may be that the question of the soul has not been relevant in your life as yet, or perhaps you have reached your conclusions. We would not wish to offer our own beliefs but to encourage you to seek your own answers in the search for total health as a 'whole being'. Practising meditation may be one way of achieving this. In the discipline of yoga, students are taught, among other things, to empty the mind of thought and free the consciousness in order to expand their understanding of the spirit. This can bring a great sense of peace and calm to those who practise the art of meditation regularly.

Environment

As an inhabitant of planet Earth, you are constantly subjected to its rhythms, moods and patterns; those you can see such as the weather and those you can't, like static electricity. Ecological events which happen in one area of the world affect people living in another. Examples such as the appalling drought in north Africa which has been linked to the destruction of vast amounts of tropical rain forest in South America, or the changing weather patterns in Europe which many believe are connected to volcano activity in North America, show us that we cannot isolate ourselves from the rest of the world.

● *Rhythms*

As with the tides, we have our own rhythms which affect the ebb and flow of energy levels. These are more obvious in women with their monthly menstrual cycle, but all humankind is subject to biological patterns governed by our own individual cycles. One obvious example of what happens when these patterns, known as circadian rhythms, go awry is jet lag. A small gland (called the pineal gland) is situated at the base of the brain. It is sensitive to light and secretes a substance known as melatonin. This, many believe, influences the pituitary gland which regulates the various levels of hormone within the body which in turn affect sleep patterns and energy levels. So when we travel very quickly from one time zone to another by jet, the body becomes confused if it feels it should be the middle of the night and yet lunch is being served!

You may be able to chart your own energy rhythms by noting when you feel more or less energetic, so that you can to some extent plan in advance when to take on tasks which are particularly demanding.

● *Air supply*

Your own personal environment is constantly affected by others, whether by something as ordinary as breathing someone else's cigarette smoke or as extraordinary as suffering the highly radioactive rainfall from the nuclear accident in Chernobyl in 1986.

It is possible to change your environment for the better. In Britain within the next few years, air should become cleaner due to the introduction of lead-free petrol. This is the result of campaigning by a group of mothers who became aware of the risks to their children's healthy development by lead pollution from petrol exhaust fumes. Lead is particularly dangerous as it affects developing cells, especially in the brain. The mental ability of children who live near busy roads has been shown to deteriorate due to lead poisoning.

Constantly inhaling polluted air will undoubtedly have a detrimental effect on your well-being. People do have to live in cities or near chemical industrial estates because of work priorities. But the risks can be minimised by taking regular trips away, especially to the coast, and also by installing air filters in your home and place of work. Filters are also very useful for the passive smoker who has either to work or live with someone who refuses to give up the deadly weed!

● *Water*

As with the air we breathe, so the water we drink is vital to our state of health. The body needs at least a couple of pints of water a day in order to function correctly, and this should be pure water in addition to other fluids. Your water supply has probably been recycled several times by the time it reaches you, causing depletion of its essential mineral content. It may also have several additions such as chlorine and fluoride. Chemicals used in farming are washed by the rain off the land and into reservoirs. In older houses, the water from your cold water tank may travel through several yards of lead piping to reach your tap. The Water Board will check your supply to tell you whether the levels of lead are safe.

To reduce these levels, ensure that when you have been on holiday and when you get up in the morning the water which has been standing in the pipes is run off without being used. never drink water from the hot tap as the heat will carry more lead with it. Water filters are available, but some of these purify to distilled standards which is not really suitable for the human body. Bottled mineral water is ideal for drinking as it usually tastes better than tap water and contains certain trace elements necessary for good health. The various spa waters contain different minerals and it is therefore better constantly to change your brand rather than stick to one.

● *Noise nuisance*

During the past 20 years, background noise levels in cities have risen dramatically. For instance, do you know of a place you can go where you will have total peace and quiet? Even in the depths of the countryside the noise of farm machinery and air traffic will probably be audible. For the most part we tend to dismiss or ignore noise, but it will still be there nagging at the unconscious and adding to stress levels. Double-glazing will reduce traffic noise levels, as will other types of insulation. Noise can be further muffled by thick fabric furnishings such as curtains and carpets which reduce echo effects. These can be particularly effective in offices where machinery causes noise nuisance.

Continuous loud noise damages the delicate workings of the inner ear. Rock musicians are often slightly deaf due to the constant assault on their ears. Personal stereo headphones can eventually have the same effect if the volume is persistently turned up high.

● *Unseen elements*

The atmosphere within which you exist contains several elements which affect the way you feel but which cannot be seen or heard. These are: temperature, humidity, ventilation, electricity and radiation. It is thought that the perfect working temperature for the brain and body is around 63°F. Any warmer and your system becomes sluggish, any cooler and you will probably feel distracted by shivering!

Ventilation is necessary to ensure that air does not become stale. If there are several people sharing one office, all breathing in the oxygen and exhaling carbon dioxide, by the end of the day the oxygen level will be fairly low. Plants absorb carbon dioxide and give out oxygen, which regulates the atmosphere perfectly. They also have the added effect of humidifying the air (as long as they are regularly watered!). A dry atmosphere will exacerbate any breathing problem or complaint of the nose and throat, the linings of which require moistness to function properly. It is possible to buy air humidifiers, but a saucer of water by a radiator is often sufficient.

It is known that before an electrical storm the atmosphere becomes charged with positive ions, which cause certain people to feel lethargic and 'muzzy headed'. Certain electrical equipment such as fluorescent lights, VDUs and televisions emit these same positive ions, creating the same effect. It is now possible to buy air ionizers which give out negative ions, thereby balancing the static electricity in the atmosphere.

Radiation is a word which strikes fear into the hearts of many and not without cause. Apart from being lethal in large doses, it speeds up the ageing process and is undoubtedly a carcinogen. Radioactivity is released into the atmosphere naturally by the sun and by certain types of rock such as granite. Tiny amounts are also discharged from some types of coal, from television screens and from luminous dials. It can also be released accidentally from nuclear power plants as happened at Chernobyl. Medical X-rays are another danger and efforts are constantly being made to reduce the levels of radiation from these without detriment to their diagnostic usefulness. Some protection can be gained against the effects on the body of radiation by taking kelp tablets which are a natural source of iodine, the substance given to radiation victims. These tablets also contain alginates which bind radioactive particles in the gut and prevent them from being absorbed into the system. Foods which contain pectin in liberal quantities, such as sunflower seeds and apples, are also helpful in preventing radiation damage to the body. They will, however, only protect the body, not heal any effects already sustained.

Achieving a balance

How balanced do you consider your life to be? All work and no play? Perhaps you are unfortunate enough to be without a job or feel the work you do is not tapping the full resources of your potential? Enduring an unsuccessful relationship within a marriage, a family or at work can cause frustration and unhappiness. Such situations create feelings of negativity and sap the energy levels. The health of the unemployed person who is understressed and bored is at as much risk as the health of the overworked and overstressed, person.

Finding a balance in your life is extremely important. If the correct balance eludes you, the temptation to resort to alcohol, cigarettes and drugs is very much greater. These substances are 'props' which artificially reduce life's pressures and make us incapable of finding solutions to our problems, thus creating a vicious circle of feelings of helplessness followed by the taking of increasing amounts of nicotine, alcohol or drugs.

Smoking

During the world wars smoking was encouraged by the governments of the time to engender feelings of comradeship. Friendships could be made by offering someone a cigarette or sharing one's last fag. Smoking also took on sexual connotations: the dim, smoky atmosphere and the act of lighting another person's cigarette were popular images portrayed in the films of the fifties. Only during the 1960s, when the effects of habitual smoking became obvious from the state of health of a generation of smokers, was it declared unhealthy.

However, by this time the taxation levied on cigarettes was a valuable source of income to governments and official anti-smoking propaganda was not forthcoming for another 10 years. During the 1970s, when unemployment started to rise, the tobacco industry was looked upon as a valuable source of employment, and so yet again the government was unwilling to put anything more than nominal pressure on smokers to give up. Horrifyingly, this is despite the fact that the cost of treating patients who have developed smoking-related diseases runs into countless millions of pounds. All of this adds weight to the argument that governments (of whatever party) do not always carry out policies which are best for the nation's health, and individuals must be responsible for themselves.

Smokers often consider lung cancer to be the only health risk they take. Smoke, of any kind, even smoked food such as kippers, may contain carcinogens (cancer-producing agents). However, apart from lung cancer, a person who smokes is also likely to die prematurely from heart disease, or from other types of cancer, bronchitis, emphysema (the destruction of lung tissue, reducing the surface area into which oxygen can be absorbed), and colitis (inflammation of the bowel, often due to the effects of nicotine). The physical effects of smoking are manifold.

As the smoke is inhaled it travels down the throat, trachea (windpipe) and on through the bronchus into the lungs. In smokers these organs are at a much higher risk of contracting cancer than in non-smokers. The smoke inhaled irritates the delicate linings of the lungs, causing them to secrete mucus, which often accounts for the typical 'smokers cough'. A tar-like deposit containing the lethal carcinogens is left in the lungs and then absorbed into the blood. Because of restricted lung actions, less oygen is admitted to the blood, giving rise to tiredness and lethargy. All the vital organs of the body are deprived of a proper supply of oxygen, thus reducing their ability to function properly. Nicotine causes the blood vessels to contract and can eventually cause the tissues in the body's extremities to be deprived of their full blood supply. These may die, become gangrenous and must be amputated.

Smokers also risk the health of those around them. 'Passive' smoking, where a non-smoker inhales another person's cigarette smoke, also increases the chances of suffering from smoking-related diseases for those who don't smoke themselves. Children will be more at risk from throat and lung infections such as tonsillitis and bronchitis, which can be extremely dangerous in very young children and babies. Asthmatic people should never live in a smoky atmosphere as this irritates their already sensitive lungs.

The health of the unborn baby is at risk from both active and passive smoking by the mother. Research in this area has shown that even the woman who regularly inhales the second-hand smoke of others runs the risk of her baby being up to five ounces lighter than normal. This can make all the difference in a baby who is already underweight due perhaps to prematurity or undernourishment from a poor placenta. Smaller babies are more prone to breathing problems.

Fortunately the non-smoking population in Britain now outnumbers those who smoke, but we still have some way to go before this is reflected in the public areas, where people are allowed to satisfy their habit. Most cinemas, trains and theatres have no-smoking areas but many restaurants have yet to follow suit. Our advice to the discontented passive smoker is to place a large notice in a prominent position stating *'No Smoking* – we are breathing today!' or 'You smoke – I choke!'

Alcohol

The consumption of alcohol is a social habit deeply entrenched in Western society – almost a way of life. Beer, spirits and wine manufacturers are, as a group, one of the most prominent users of advertising, capitalising on people's subconscious wish to fit into a certain group, whether it be 'one of the lads' or the sophisticated jetsetter. Alcoholic drink is also to be seen in television serials, plays and films. The social pressures to drink are enormous and often subliminal, so great is the exposure, but the human cost in misery and suffering cannot be estimated.

Dependency upon alcohol becomes dangerous as soon as the person concerned feels he or she cannot get by without a drink even when the quantity is relatively small, although obviously the larger the amount the greater the risk to health. Because of their smaller size and slower metabolism, women are at greater risk than men. There is no getting away from the fact that alcohol is a poison and a drug. But what exactly are the risks?

The liver is the organ most likely to be affected by heavy drinking and the one most people readily associate with alcoholism. Cirrhosis of the liver develops over a number of years leading to enlargement and hardening of this vital organ, subsequently leading to jaundice and inability to purify the blood properly. Poisons normally excreted from the body are absorbed into the blood. The chances of developing cancer of some part of the digestive tract (mouth, throat, stomach and intestines) are increased in even relatively light drinkers, as are disorders of the kidneys and bladder. Alcohol causes dehydration of the system, the effects of which are most readily seen in the skin which needs moisture to stay firm and supple. Deprived of its supply of moisture, the skin can become prematurely wrinkled. The body's vitamin supply is also depleted to the detriment of those organs which need vitamins to function correctly.

Despite all this there is no doubt that alcohol is here to stay and one would have to be a complete killjoy to ban it altogether. But some measures can be taken to minimise the risks. As a general rule, no more than two units of alcohol should be drunk in any one day. (A unit equals half a pint of beer, or one measure of spirits, or one glass of wine.) Alcohol should never be drunk on an empty stomach as it is then absorbed directly through the stomach wall into the bloodstream. Rice and pasta are excellent foods to eat beforehand as these will absorb some of the alcohol thereby protecting the stomach lining. The dehydrating effects can be avoided to some extent by alternating each alcoholic drink with a glass of water. If alcohol is taken regularly, it is advisable to take multivitamin tablets in order to avoid becoming vitamin deficient.

Drugs

Although both nicotine and alcohol are drugs in their own right, the term 'drugs' tends to be used separately to describe substances which are prescribed for medicinal purposes, or obtained illegally for their ability artificially to induce a particular state of mind and body. All drugs, even the humblest aspirin, should be taken with caution and treated with respect for their usage.

Over the past 20 years or so the tranquilliser has probably been the most misused of all drugs. It has been seen as a cure-all for mental and emotional problems as well as associated physical disorders. Many people exist with dulled senses, living a slow-motion life. This does not take into account those who are addicted to illegal substances whose effects are seen all too frequently and tragically. It is sad but true that many people 'would rather die than think', as Bertrand Russell once said. Recent medical evidence has shown that such drugs can be carcinogens, particularly if taken on a regular, long-term basis. However, weaning off their tablets patients who have reached the stage of addiction is a delicate process requiring support and encouragement through the withdrawal stage and after. Patients need to find some way of coping with life and its associated stresses.

Get organised

An organised life seems to be the key to successful modern living. It is possible to gain control of one's life and to expend energies in the areas where they are most required. This can only be achieved once these key areas are identified and understood. Only you as an individual know what your greatest needs in life are and where your hopes lie.

All too often fear of failure is translated into 'not having the time' to attempt to carry out a certain task. Mental energy is wasted on thought processes which are disorganised and confused. Supposing you are busy, with many tasks to complete within a certain time span. If you do not allocate a certain length of time for each task, you are likely to feel panic as you worry that each job will not be completed in time. The rising panic levels destroy your concentration on the task in hand and lead to poor standards of work with, in the long run, a lessening of self-esteem. Sickness can also be an 'avoidance technique' when the mind translates the fear of an event into genuine illness.

Becoming organised will take time and effort. Examine the way you spend your time at present and reallocate it to your advantage. Start by writing down all the key areas in your life on which you spend your time. It may take you a while to do this as there will be all sorts of details which don't immediately spring to mind. Prepare a list of headings such as work, leisure, family, friends, eating, sleeping, travelling, shopping, domestic duties – all those which apply to your life. (If you use public transport, you will probably be surprised at how much of your time you spend travelling or waiting for trains and buses to arrive.)

Under each main heading list related activities. For example, the heading 'family' might contain a list of relations, such as spouse, children, parents, brother, granny, aunt, whom you see throughout the year. Next to each write down the time you actually spend with each and then consider whether this is too much or not enough. Now consider what is the ideal amount of time you prefer to spend with each and write that down next to the actual times. Remember, this is your own private exercise so there is no need to feel guilty if there is someone you would rather see less often.

When you are satisfied that you have gathered all the information on how you spend your time, transfer it into a chart and it will help you to see your life as a whole rather than as a series of fragmented activities. As much as a third of your time may be spent sleeping. Now do the same with the second list of *preferred* time spent on the same activities and compare the two charts. Aim to achieve a balance between work, leisure activities and relaxation, ensuring that at least as much time is given to doing things you enjoy as to those you don't.

To complete this exercise, write down all your expectations of life, your dreams and ambitions. Let your imagination run wild, this is for your eyes only. Choose the item on this list which you would most like to achieve and make time each week to get a little nearer to your goal, whatever it is!

Now that you have a set of goals and a plan of how you would prefer to spend your time, you can start to work towards them. Aim to be as realistic as possible, using the knowledge you have of your own personality. For instance, if you are a night owl who has difficulty rising early in the morning, don't start by aiming to begin the day at six o'clock! Begin organising your time by making out a plan for the coming week, month, year and even five years. List all the activities you wish to carry out during that period and then assess at the end of the time span whether you have managed to achieve all, some or none. Try not to become discouraged if you have not managed to accomplish all the tasks you have set yourself. Perhaps your expectations of yourself (or someone else) were too high. Readjust the allotted time accordingly. Remember to take into account your own periods of high and low energy output. Lastly, and most

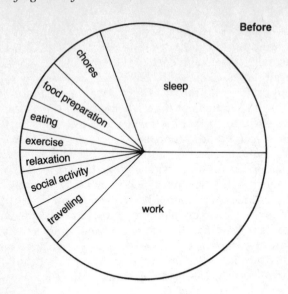

Before

Plan your day:

Before *Too much time is spent sleeping and too much on chores. Decide to get up earlier, do essential chores first thing. Take more exercise.*

important, do not forget to spend the time you put aside to achieve your dream goal on doing just that!

Holidays

Apart from the aforementioned 'props', another way of alleviating the rigorous pressures of living is to take a holiday. The tourist industry is a multimillion pound business, the sole aim of which is to lure us out of our normal routines to spend our hard-earned cash on travelling to a different place in which to pass our leisure time. Perhaps the boom in this industry over the past 20 years shows only too clearly the need in our society to 'get away from it all'. Very enjoyable it can be too, except that it is often the case that one set of stresses is swapped for another. During the darkest days of winter when the sun barely makes an appearance and

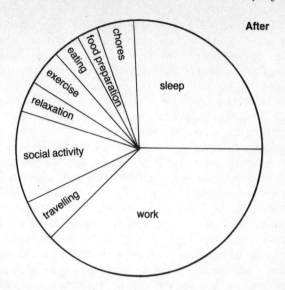

After

chores

food preparation

eating

exercise

relaxation

social activity

travelling

sleep

work

After More time is available for social activities. Food preparation time has been reduced by changing to healthier, less-elaborate meals.

Each circle represents 24 hours. You can do the same for a week, a month or a year.

depression is rife, the glossy brochures are a promise of better times ahead. Unfortunately, the fact that we are all too ready to have our expectations of the perfect holiday raised to ridiculously high levels leaves us susceptible to disappointment.

There is no doubt that those who live in less sunny climes are prone to depression from lack of the golden rays. This depression may have a physical basis due to the activity of the light-sensitive pineal gland mentioned already. It is thought that this gland secretes hormones which improve our mood and make us feel happier. If we are deprived of sunshine, the gland is not activated and we are miserable. It would seem that those races which live in darkness for six months of the year, such as Eskimoes, are far better able to adjust to their sunshine deficiency.

So, the majority of us look forward to our annual sunshine break, and if the weather isn't perfect every day for the fourteen or however many days of our holiday, frustration ensues. These feelings are entirely due to our expectations being dashed. We feel the same if it doesn't snow on a skiing holiday or if the wind doesn't blow for a sailing holiday. Perhaps Holiday Rule Number One should read: Ban all expectations to avoid disappointment.

Should our prayers be answered and the sun shine brilliantly and constantly, then the risks to the health of the fair-skinned become greater. The incidence of skin cancer (melanoma) has increased greatly over the past few years. This seems to be related to the growth in popularity of sunbathing and acquiring a suntan. The people most at risk from melanoma are those with an Irish/Scottish type of skin which tends to be white with freckles. Short, sharp bursts of sunshine seem to be the most dangerous type of exposure, especially if one becomes sunburnt. However, if skin cancer is treated in its early stages there is a good chance of survival. Any brown pigmentation, such as a mole, should be watched for any sign of change in shape, colour or size. Bleeding, itchy patches which appear for no apparent reason should never be ignored. The more moles a person has, the higher the risk of contracting skin cancer. Those people with very fair skins should forget about trying to acquire a tan and attempt instead to be pale and interesting.

Even those with darker skins need to make careful use of sun filters and stay indoors between the hours of 11 am and 2 pm when the sun is at its strongest. Remember also that the sun's ultraviolet rays travel through water and are reflected from its surface. Protection from these rays is also necessary when sitting in the shade as the rays are still being reflected into shady areas. Therefore, Holiday Rule Number Two is: Take care in the sun.

The holiday season is also traditionally a family time when partners, their offspring, and sometimes other relatives, gather to spend their leisure time together. After the initial mood of *bonhomie* has subsided, relationships which have usually survived on fairly limited contact come under pressure. When the partners in a shaky relationship are thrown together for a period of continual contact, then the problems become less easy to hide or avoid. Confrontation is almost inevitable. Holidays do not usually cause a crisis within a relationship, but can certainly highlight one. Differences of opinion over how to spend the time, where to go and who disciplines the kids are all symptoms of deeper underlying problems which may need sorting out.

These problems can be shelved to some extent until after the holiday, when an attempt can be made to solve them. However, a chilly atmosphere can ruin a good holiday and is hardly conducive to relaxation. If as a rule the members of a family spend very little time together, a long spell of enforced company can feel claustrophobic. People begin to feel guilty that they resent the presence of the others around them, and this adds to feelings of unease.

Allowing space for yourself and other people, rather than expecting everyone to get along marvellously for a whole fortnight, can alleviate this problem to some degree. If you go away with friends, make sure you have separate living accommodation and have a set of ground rules such as sharing any chores and, more importantly, agreeing to go your separate ways when there is a difference of opinion over a particular suggested activity or excursion. Many are the friendships which have foundered on the rocks of joint holidays. Holiday Rule Number Three must be: Allow space for each individual to be themselves rather than the person you think they should be.

The digestive system is likely to suffer upset on holiday. It is abused by strange food and water, and by excess alcohol, and is jiggled around with nerves and excitement. It is hardly surprising that it often fails to work properly and diarrhoea and vomiting result. Given a choice, our stomachs would probably rather stay at home. Holiday tummy upsets are seldom due to a specific infection or food poisoning. The most usual cause for the 'Spanish Squits', 'Delhi Belly' and 'Roman Runs' is the local water supply. Even when this is deemed safe to drink, it is far more sensible to drink only bottled mineral water. The problem is the different mineral components of local water rather than pollution. Your system would become used to it in time. Likewise with the local food; gradually introduce the more exotic dishes during the holiday and give your stomach time to adjust. Shellfish are a particular cause of food poisoning, and those varieties which are eaten raw, such as oysters, have been found to cause hepatitis – so be warned.

In order to give your stomach a chance to stay healthy on holiday, you can fortify its immune system in advance. The gut contains bacteria which fight off any infection, and this action can be effectively strengthened by eating 'live' yoghurt which contains similar bacteria. A couple of spoonfuls per day is adequate. Another useful aid to digestion is garlic which can be taken in the form of 'perles' which guarantee no aftertaste. These capsules should be taken for two weeks before departure and also during the holiday. *Never*, *ever* take antibiotics when suffering from diarrhoea and vomiting as these will destroy the helpful bacteria and ultimately delay your recovery. Always check with your GP several weeks before you leave as to whether vaccinations for typhoid and cholera are necessary, especially if you are going somewhere exotic. Holiday Rule Number Four is therefore: Give your stomach some thought.

Organising in advance, with preparation for possible hitches, can alleviate some of the stresses of travelling to distant climes. This can be done without making it seem too much like a military campaign! If you know that you have adequate insurance cover for medical bills or car repairs you have less to worry about when these happen. Keep all your valuables and spare cash in the hotel safe and carry an appropriate credit card, so that if your money and travellers' cheques are stolen you are not completely destitute. Remember to pack a comprehensive first aid kit containing all those preparations you use regularly at home, and include insect repellent along with something for treating bites and stings. A useful tip for packing is to put some clothing for each member of the travelling party into each case and take some toiletries in your handluggage. Then when you are in Rimini and one stray suitcase has gone to Dubai, everyone will at least have a change of clothing.

If you are taking young children on holiday, remember to take a large supply of wet cleaning tissues, new books or comics and their favourite soft toys. You will find it much easier to settle a small child in a strange bedroom if he or she has something familiar to hold. Finally, if you take children plan the whole event around them with activities organised for each part of the day. This is the only way you will get any peace. (It has taken us eight years to discover this!) Holiday rule Number Five, then? Thorough organisation will help to relieve stress.

Safety

Throughout life certain chances have to be taken in order to make progress. For many people risk is the piquant sauce of life and without it things can become very boring. However, risks are best taken with full knowledge of the situation, in order to minimise the possible dangerous consequences. For example, the parachutist will not take to the air without full training, a correctly packed parachute, and a second one in case the first fails. Minimising the risk of accident means being fully aware of the dangers, and enables you to take measures to counteract them.

Accidents are far more likely to happen if we are not in good health. We tend to think of accidents happening on the roads, in factories and on construction sites, whereas in fact the majority happen within our homes, paradoxically the place we feel safest. Hospital casualty departments are continually dealing with burns, scalds, cuts and broken bones sustained mainly by improper use of equipment and carelessness at home. The young and old in our society are most at risk from accidents which, by their very nature, might have been prevented with a little forethought.

The state of our health has great bearing on how accident-prone we are. It is a well-documented fact that women who suffer from pre-menstrual syndrome are more likely to have accidents at this time during their cycle. As many as two-thirds of all road accidents involve people who have consumed alcohol, which slows down reflexes and causes erratic behaviour. If you are tired, in a hurry or under stress then you are likely to be preoccupied and, therefore, less careful than usual in your actions. A number of serious diseases are likely to cause clumsiness in their initial stages. These include muscular dystrophy, multiple sclerosis, Parkinson's disease and occasionally brain tumours.

● *The elderly.* This group of people are most at risk from falls, poisoning and burns. As they are often unsteady on their feet and suffer from poor eyesight, an uneven step, the edge of a rug or a frayed piece of carpet can be a major hazard. Poor lighting adds to the risk. As many as 3,000 people (most of them elderly) die each year as a result of falling. Often it is not their injuries which kill them but pneumonia which attacks because they are immobile and in a weak and shocked condition.

Old people these days are frequently prescribed a large number of tablets. (Anecdote from Mike: 'I once knew an old chap who had been prescribed a total of no less than 16 different tablets. He kept them altogether in a sweetie jar and took the first dozen which came out each morning!') No doubt confused by their usage, elderly people will often forget which tablets they have already taken and what is the correct dosage. Also, it is unfortunately true that they are prescribed doses of drugs which are far too large for their systems to cope with. This frequently leads to accidental poisoning.

Attempts to keep warm create further accidents. Old electric blankets constitute a particular hazard. The bedclothes may ignite by coming into contact with a frayed flex, or the person forgets to switch off the blanket before getting into bed and perhaps spills a drink. Many deaths from burns occur because of the lethal habit of smoking in bed.

Over-enthusiastic attempts to keep out draughts may result in carbon dioxide poisoning. This occurs when the fire burns up all the oxygen supply in a badly ventilated room. Sadly, the flip side of this situation is that often inadequate heating causes hypothermia and people die from the cold. Every year brings news of several old people who have died from this condition during a cold spell. Hypothermia is a gradual condition where people will initially feel cold, then lethargic, and eventually slip into unconsciousness. If they are not found in time, death will result. Should you ever find a person suffering from hypothermia it is important to remember to bring the body temperature back to normal slowly. Administer warm (not hot) drinks and cover with blankets whilst waiting for the emergency services to arrive.

● *Children*. As many as a quarter of all accidents involving children occur in other people's homes. For example, 20,000 of the 80,000 garden accidents happen whilst on a visit to a friend or relative. This would seem to be mainly due to the place being unfamiliar territory and the fact that the people visited are unused to having children about and are unaware of the dangers. Parents are often less vigilant with their children when visiting as they are preoccupied with being sociable guests.

Supervision of children is often reduced when a parent is ill or has to look after another sick child. If there is a new baby, the mother tends to be more tired and occupied than usual and the older child will often try to gain the parents' attention by doing things it knows are forbidden.

Children are constantly at risk from poisoning. Grandparents' tablets, bleaches or chemicals left around in accessible places are often a temptation, especially if they are in containers which look similar to lemonade bottles or sweet jars. Try to teach your children from a very early age not to eat anything from the garden without asking an adult first.

When a child first starts to walk about, the parents are often not familar with the safety hazards which abound in the home, particularly if it is their first child. Having been used to an immobile little bundle, it is a major upheaval to be one step ahead of a lively toddler who sees the world as a great adventure. Burns and scalds are some of the most horrific accidents to happen in the home, particularly to the very young child who pulls a tablecloth, along with the teapot, on to itself. Irons, kettles and electric sockets are also dangerous objects to this age group.

Five thousand children each year are seriously, sometimes fatally, injured in accidents involving glass doors. A particular hazard is the glass-panelled door at the foot of the stairs or hallway – a favourite play area for children. More recently, large patio doors have become popular in homes. When these are unmarked, children (and adults) have been known to walk straight through them, causing appalling injuries.

To err is human and we all make mistakes, but the very nature of accidents means that with some forethought the majority of them could have been prevented. By becoming aware of the risks you might spare yourself serious injury, debility and a guilty conscience for the rest of your life.

2
A dictionary of alternative therapies

With the growth in use and popularity of 'natural methods' of healing over the past few years, many complementary and alternative therapies have come into practice, some of which are new and others of which are thousands of years old. This chapter is an outline guide to what they are and how they are used.

The list is for your information rather than for specific recommendations. When seeking help with a health problem from an alternative or complementary practitioner, always endeavour to visit a trained and registered person. For example, if you wish to visit an osteopath, find one who is a member of the Register of Osteopaths. Whenever possible, try to use one who has been personally recommended. All good practitioners abhor the 'quacks' who set themselves up without adequate training or knowledge, bringing the service into disrepute.

A final word of warning. The body needs time to heal, but simple conditions should improve within a few weeks. If they do not or if they become worse, then it is unlikely that the treatment is doing you any good and may possibly even be harmful. Never forget that you are an individual and, as such, need treatment tailored to your needs. What has helped another person may not necessarily help you.

Acupressure Using the same meridians as acupuncture, this method uses the application of pressure rather than puncturing the skin with a needle. Used for the same conditions as acupuncture.

Acupuncture This ancient Chinese art involves placing fine metal needles (pure copper, gold or silver may be used) into specific points along the meridians of the body. These meridians are thought of as energy channels, and the placing of needles into them sets up a current which passes via the central nervous system into the corresponding organ. Acupuncturists believe that if the organ is imbalanced and therefore sick, the imbalance can be corrected by this technique. The needles are not inserted too deeply into the skin and should cause very little discomfort if treatment is practised by an experienced acupuncturist.

The Chinese often burn herbal leaves on the ends of the needles to increase the efficacy of the current. In Britain, a mild electric current is sometimes passed through the needles to obtain the same effect.

Although it can be used as a curative form of therapy for many illnesses, acupuncture is most useful for the relief of chronic pain. In its purest form the true Chinese acupuncturist will use it in conjunction with diet to *prevent* illness occurring, which is why, traditionally, patients would pay only when they were well.

Alexander technique Based on the methods formulated and used by Frederick Matthias Alexander who died in London in 1955, this therapy involves teaching the patient the 'correct usage' of muscle groups and posture. Poor posture can create tension in muscles, which may eventually cause diseases. A practitioner of Alexander's methods will correct postural faults, thereby relieving muscle tension and allowing the free use of muscle groups.

Used in particular for those ailments which have their root cause in muscle tension and misalignment of joints such as fibrositis, arthritis, slipped disc and back problems.

Aromatherapy This technique uses massage to apply a range of essential oils to the skin. These oils are the pure, concentrated essences of a variety of fragrant plants such as tuberose and geranium. The various oils are absorbed through the skin and the aromas are inhaled, producing a range of therapeutic effects to relax or invigorate the subject into whom they are rubbed.

Used mainly as a treatment for stress.

Art therapy The art therapist encourages his or her clients to use different artistic media (paint, chalk, clay etc.) as a means of expression of the client's innermost feelings. The aim is to work through emotional problems about which it is difficult to talk openly.

Used especially for those people suffering emotional upset who find it difficult to communicate with words alone.

Auras Certain people believe they are able to see a light/energy field surrounding human beings which gives information relating to a person's personality and state of well-being. It is thought that the halos portrayed around Christ and the saints are related to this particular practice.

Auricular therapy This involves the placing of needles into the channels which run through the ear, and is a form of acupuncture. All the organs of the body may be mapped out within the ear, which is believed to correspond to the shape of a human foetus.

Bach's flower remedies Based on the work of Dr Edward Bach (born 1886), who became disillusioned with contemporary orthodox medicine and worked out a system using non-poisonous herbs for remedial purposes, often using himself as a guinea pig for his experiments.

His treatments are used in conjunction with a diagnosis of the patient's emotional state. Bach classified these states into seven main categories including depression, isolation and negativity, and used different flowers or herbs to treat the different conditions. For example, he would treat with honeysuckle those who suffered because of yearning nostalgically for the past.

Biofeedback This is a diagnostic method which uses a special instrument to record changes in the body's pulses in order to detect physical disorders. The patient has wires attached which feed into a monitor that gives a reading indicating the state of health. This reading is, in turn, interpreted by the therapist. Biofeedback is often used in the detection of allergies.

Biomagnetics A system claiming, by the use of magnets placed at strategic points on the body, to balance the magnetic polarity of the body which, if disturbed, can make the patient feel unwell and less resistant to illness.

Chelation A method of 'cleaning out' the arteries of the body which have become clogged by atheroma, the substance responsible for the hardening of the arteries which can lead to possible strokes and heart attacks. A synthetic amino acid known as EDTA is dripped into the patient's bloodstream where it binds together the dangerous minerals which constitute atheroma. These are then excreted from the body.

Used for patients known to suffer from the effects of 'furred-up' arteries, such as stroke and heart patients.

Chiropractic A therapy based on the belief that all the systems of the body rely upon good alignment of the muscular-skeletal frame, in particular the spine. A chiropractor will manoeuvre the bones into the correct position and use massage to aid the healing process.

Used particularly for back problems and neuralgia.

Chromatherapy A method of healing using coloured light. Colour therapists base their treatments on the belief that each of the body's 'chakras' (energy centres also used in yoga) is governed by a particular colour. The patient's body is bathed in the appropriate coloured light or the patient may be given training in colour visualisation to obtain the desired healing effect.

Herbalism The very oldest form of medicine known to humankind has always been used very widely throughout the underdeveloped world. Herbs and mixtures of herbs are known to have curative effects, and many modern medicines are derived from them.

Formal training in herbal medicine is now increasingly available in developed societies and practitioners will carefully prescribe medicines that are preventative and curative.

Holistic practitioner A person whose treatments are based on the view of the 'whole' person, rather than just the disease. This type of practitioner will take into account the balance of the patient's emotional, physical, mental and spiritual conditions before prescribing a relevant therapy.

Homeopathy Originating in Germany in the late eighteenth century, this method of treatment is the alternative which has found most favour with orthodox medical opinion. It is based on the belief that a minute dose of the substance which has caused the disease of the body will stimulate the 'vital force' to promote healing. The practice is very much based on treatment of the person rather than the disease.

Hydrotherapy A form of cure using water, usually cold or alternating the application of hot and cold water. High-powered jets of water are sometimes used in order to stimulate the blood circulation in a specific part of the body. Spa baths are a popular form of treatment for arthritis sufferers. The patient is immersed in water containing minerals said to be beneficial in the cure of this type of disease. Some types of physiotherapy are carried out in a pool in order to relieve the patient of the weight of the body, so that exercise is easier to perform.

Hypnotherapy Hypnotism is another complementary practice which is often carried out by orthodox physicians. A hypnotist will enable the patient to induce a trance-like state which can be of varying depth. The patient is able to respond to the practitioner and also to remember what has happened during the trance. It is said that no one can be hypnotised against their will. Little is known about how or why it works, but the effects are more beneficial when the patient is completely relaxed and has a measure of trust in the hypnotist. It is often used for the treatment of phobias, to relieve the pain of childbirth and to help patients give up smoking.

Iridology A method of diagnosing illness before it becomes otherwise apparent in the person by 'reading' the eye. The practitioner believes that the organs of the body can be mapped out in the eye and that any spots, marks or cracks in certain areas predict trouble for the corresponding organ of the body.

Kinesiology Another oriental-based practice using the scientific study of human movement which is thought to be related to disease. Massage and postural changes are used to aid the healing process.

Massage A widely used method of alleviating muscular tension by the application of firm but gentle pressure to an affected part of the body (see also page 72).

Naturopathy Also known as 'nature cure', this is another form of treatment of the 'whole person'. There are two schools of thought: one which is purist (using only diet, exercise and massage) the other using these in conjunction with some of the other aforementioned complementary techniques such as acupuncture and homeopathy.

Osteopathy This system of healing uses massage and manipulation in order to relieve the pain which arises from bruising or displacement of the muscular-skeletal frame. The method is particularly used for problems relating to the spine, which contains the central nervous system, and for arthritis sufferers in order to ease and mobilise their stiff joints.

Psychotherapy A method of healing emotional wounds by examining and 'working through' feelings which the patient finds difficult to cope with. This is an intrinsic part of holistic healing, as negative emotions which are not dealt with are often part and parcel of a physical illness.

Radionics This practice is based on the ancient technique of 'dowsing' or 'divining' which is better known as a technique for finding water or precious metals. Certain individuals are thought to be able to detect illness by holding a pendulum or metal rod or perhaps a lock of their hair near to the patient. The way in which the pendulum swings or the rod twitches is interpreted by the therapist in order to diagnose an illness or allergy.

Rebirthing Therapists who use this method of treatment believe that a difficult birth process results in trauma for the baby causing psychological and often physical illness in later life. The process involves hyperventilation (deep, rapid breathing) and reliving the birth in a supposedly more gentle and controlled manner.

Reflexology Therapists using this particular form of therapy believe that the organs of the body can be mapped out on the soles of the feet. If an organ is diseased then the corresponding part of the foot may feel sore and, to the reflexologist, 'gritty' to the touch. The feet are methodically massaged, as in acupressure, in order to stimulate healing.

Regression Some therapists use hypnosis in order to get patients to relive a traumatic experience which occurred at an earlier stage in their life and has lain buried in the memory because of its painful associations, causing illness and even psychosis. There is a school of thought which believes people can be regressed into a former life.

Reichian therapy Austrian-born William Reich (1897–1957) formulated the theory that mental and emotional stresses are unconsciously expressed in the body. By massaging particular muscle groups, tension which relates to previous traumas that has been held for some time in the subconscious, may be released in the form of emotions. Once released, these feelings can then be examined and resolved by discussion. This therapy is usually carried out within a group situation.

Spiritual healing Healers of this type believe that they can channel the universal force of energy which emanates from God, in order to promote healing in others. This may be done in the time-honoured way by the 'laying on of hands' or by visualising the sick person at a distance, possibly using a photograph or lock of hair belonging to the patient.

Touch for health This therapy involves both diagnosis and healing by the method of muscle-testing based on kinesiology. Treatment of an affected part is carried out by massage. These therapists also believe that allergy to certain foods can be detected by testing whether a muscle becomes weaker when an allergenic substance is placed close to the patient's body.

Transcutaneous nerve stimulation (TNS) This is a method of relieving pain by the use of a small, battery-operated machine attached to the patient's affected part by means of electrodes. An electronic pulse is given by the machine to the patient, stimulating the body's own endorphins or pain-killing hormones. One use is to relieve pain during childbirth.

Visualisation Patients using this type of therapy are first taught deep relaxation techniques. When relaxed they are asked to visualise the affected part of their body and use imagery to promote its return to health. For example, the patient may use the thought of the good cells fighting a winning battle against the diseased cells.

3
Food and diet

There is perhaps no better way to demonstrate the respect you feel for yourself than through your choice of food and the manner in which you consume it. A person with a poor self-image may be obese or, conversely, anorexic. Such people translate their feelings about themselves into physical terms either by compulsive eating, risking all the attendant health problems of obesity or, in the case of the anorexic, by starving, in some cases to death.

Food is the fuel which determines whether we run smoothly on all four cylinders or career around backfiring, spluttering and eventually slowing to a halt. Our eating habits are inextricably linked to our emotions. From the moment the umbilical cord is cut we are dependent on the love and care of others, usually our mothers, to feed us, in order that we may survive. Throughout childhood food is used by some parents as a means of showing care in place of emotional sustenance. Thus children quickly learn to use their eating habits to demonstrate feelings of anger by rejecting food given by a parent, or to gain attention by poor behaviour at the table and becoming a 'fussy eater'. Parents who insist that their children eat huge amounts of food (this being their way of showing love) thus create feelings of guilt in a child who finds it difficult to finish the portions. These feelings are often transferred into adult relationships and continue into the next generation. Obese people often eat to 'comfort' themselves.

Food is our third most important need after air and water; without it we would eventually die. This importance, along with the pleasure we derive from satisfying our appetites, has put eating at the centre of our daily lives. Food also has great social and religious significance. It follows that inadequate or unsuitable food is going to cause problems. Of course, there are many stages along the road to poor nutrition before starvation point is reached. For instance, deficient or unbalanced meals are eaten by many apparently wealthy nations, resulting in poor health. If you feel generally unwell and frequently suffer from illness, you should examine your diet before any other area of your lifestyle, such is its importance to your well-being.

Since World War 2 our foods have become increasingly refined, sugary and high in fat content. Chemicals have been introduced to preserve, colour and flavour foods in order to prolong their 'shelf life' and entice us to buy them. These movements in the food industry have seemingly led to a high incidence of heart disease, allergies and cancer. In fact, a poor diet may be partly responsible for the destruction of the immune system, illness always being at least partially rooted in poor eating habits. Those people who have opted for a healthier, wholefood diet will testify to the improvement felt in their health within a short time span. The wish to become healthier and the effort you take to feed your body the correct foodstuffs will give you some of the positive messages required to remain fit and well.

So how do you decide what is healthy food and what is not? Where do you begin? It is very difficult to decide what you are doing wrong until you know exactly what your diet consists of. For a week, write down everything you eat and drink including the time at which you consume it. Also, note down the periods of the day when you feel tired or edgy and those at which you feel your most energetic.

Eating habits are almost as important as the type of food you eat. You are aiming for a balanced, varied diet, high in fibre, low in fat, rich in vitamins and minerals and with only small amounts of sugar, salt and artificial additives.

The level of your intake of stimulants such as caffeine, alcohol and nicotine should also be taken into consideration. Note which substances you reach for when you are under stress. A cigarette, a cup of coffee or an alcoholic drink? You may find you are attracted to sweet foods when you feel pressured. Whatever the substance, that is likely to be the one to which your system has become addicted. If this is the case, then you are likely to go through a period of craving once you cut out that particular element.

● *Food sensitivities.*
In recent years food allergies have become more widely accepted as a cause of ill-health. It is not an easy task to discover what is causing the allergy, although you may undergo tests to pinpoint the particular culprit in your diet.

The most common foodstuffs which cause allergies are coffee, cheese, milk, wheat and chocolate, along with a range of chemical food additives. If you suffer from headaches, lethargy or rashes then it may be that you are allergic to a food you eat regularly as part of your normal diet. Under the supervision of your doctor you will need to cleanse your system by fasting and then introduce foods gradually until you find the particular one which is causing your ill-health. Alternatively, if you consider one type of food to be suspect, cut it out of your diet for a week and see if you improve.

● *Happy shopping habits.*
Have a look through your cupboards so that you know what your shopping habits are. Do you have packets of instant, chemical-loaded foods and sugary snacks such as cakes, biscuits and sweets? How many pieces of fresh fruit and vegetables do you have? Take a look at the tins and packets and read the labels.

With the trend towards healthier food, manufacturers now often label food 'natural', but this often doesn't mean an awful lot. Snack bars which are advertised as being 'full of goodness, containing syrup, glucose and chocolate' may often be read as actually containing sugar, sugar and sugar! Even so-called 'health bars' are suspect in this regard. The most innocent-looking foods, such as breakfast cereals, are 'doctored' with sugar and salt. Packet soups are real offenders here. Many are chemical cocktails with the smallest amount of asparagus or chicken added at the end of the list! Another endearing trick employed by food manufacturers is to label prominently the fact that their food has no added artificial flavourings or colourings. Small print will then state that it is loaded with sugar and preservatives. Endeavour to become an habitual label reader when you are shopping for food so that you develop healthy habits. If your cupboards do not contain rubbish then you can't eat it!

Before you commence your healthier diet, consider and write down the reasons why you are doing this. To lessen your risk of developing a serious disease? So that you might feel generally healthier? To lose weight? Know what you are aiming at so that you can chart your progress. If you are feeling low, this is not a good time to be attempting a change. You will return to the old bad habits quickly and will feel twice the failure for it, confirming your own worst suspicions about yourself. Do not underestimate how closely your eating habits are linked to your psyche.

What is 'a healthy diet'?

The word 'diet' has been synonymous, in our generally overfed society, with an attempt to lose weight. In fact people who eat a nutritionally balanced diet (high in fibre, rich in fresh foods, low in fat, sugar and salt) never have the need to go on a reducing diet as their weight remains steady at the *correct level for them*. People who eat a poor, overly refined diet need to eat far more food to meet the nutritional needs of their bodies. This means that when they try to eat less of the same poor-quality foodstuffs, in order to lose weight, they feel deprived and 'starved'.

Sugar is a very quick source of energy. You may find that when you are hungry you crave sweet food (though what you need is protein). However, sugar is empty of nutritional value, so when that energy is used up the deeper nutritional needs of the body have not been met. This pattern may eventually set up a sugar addiction, believed by some medical and alternative practitioners to endanger the immune system, causing the body to become vulnerable to disease and, of course, leading to extra body weight. Yeast-based fungal

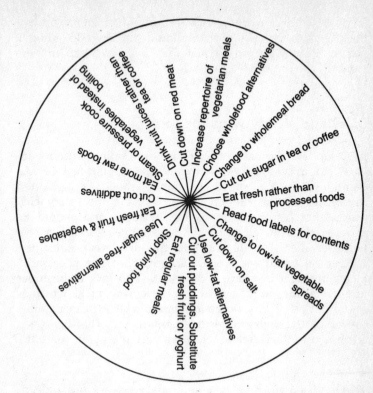

A healthy-eating wheel. Choose any starting-point. Make one change per week.

infections, such as thrush, thrive on sugars. These problems are in addition to the well-documented side-effect of tooth decay.

A diet which contains the correct vitamins and minerals along with fibre, carbohydrate, protein and a small amount of fat allows the body to function correctly in a healthy manner. Fluids are of equal nutritional importance to food. Water helps to flush out the system and should be drunk throughout the day. Fresh fruit juices also help to cleanse the system of impurities and contain vitamins. Coffee, tea, chocolate and other such beverages should be kept to a minimum due to their containing caffeine, sugar or fat. In order not to disrupt the digestive process, drinks should be taken 15 minutes before or after a meal so that the juices excreted into the stomach are not diluted.

Slow and steady wins the race

Any sudden, dramatic changes in your eating patterns are likely to upset your system and make you feel ill. As mentioned in the previous chapter, holidays are often responsible for this sudden change, causing upset stomachs. This is not conducive to feeling healthier and should be avoided. Set yourself a plan for a week-by-week change to a healthier diet. For instance, in the first week substitute wholemeal bread for white. 'Brown' does not necessarily mean healthier as some bread is dyed to give a 'healthier hue'. It is the bran content in wholemeal bread which is important as dietary fibre. In some of the African nations, cancer of the colon is virtually unknown. This has been attributed to their diet which has a very high bran content.

● *Fibre.*
This has been much talked about in recent times and, indeed, it is important in that the bowels need bulk in order to stimulate the wave-like peristaltic action of the muscles which move the waste products out of your body. Fibre also holds excess carbohydrate in the gut so that it is not absorbed into the system and laid down as fat cells. As you get older, fibre becomes more important in this cleansing and stimulating process.

If you are trying to educate your whole family into healthier eating habits, it may be necessary to introduce the new products slowly over a period of time, gradually weaning the family off the less nutritious items and on to the wholefood alternatives. For example, you may introduce wholewheat pasta and brown rice in preference to the refined 'white' version.

● *Salt*.

If you use salt on your food and in your cooking, gradually cut down the amount. The taste change can be tempered by flavouring with other spices. Too much salt means that body fluid is retained instead of being excreted through the kidneys. This leads to a bloated feeling. Many naturopaths believe that a salty diet hinders the healing process in the body. Medical evidence has shown that in some patients it is responsible for causing high blood pressure in later life. Aim towards refraining from sprinkling salt on food if it has been used during cooking, and remove the cruet from the table for good! If you use stock cubes, do not add extra salt to the dish as most proprietary brands are high in salt content. Remember, it's not just the salt that you see, such as that sprinkled on potato crisps, it is also the salt which you don't see that destroys, for example hard cheese is quite high in salt content. Once again, read the label!

● *Fats*.

These are stored in the body to be converted into energy should there be no easier supply available in the form of sugar or carbohydrate. If you have excess body fat which you wish to be rid of, then it is necessary to have a diet containing very little fat or carbohydrate and no sugar. Under these conditions your body will use up the store of fats available to it.

This, however, should be a slow process due to the fact that lean (muscle) tissue is lost twice as quickly as fat. Consider that your heart is made up of lean muscle and you will understand why it is necessary to go very slowly when on a reducing diet if you are not to weaken your heart. Steady exercise such as swimming, cycling or jogging should be taken during this period to build up lean muscle tissue and to use up energy. You will then avoid the trap which many dieters fall into, known as the Yo-Yo syndrome, when a large amount of weight is lost very quickly on a strict low-calorie diet and then regained as soon as a normal diet is resumed.

It is also thought in some quarters that toxins absorbed into the body, from pollution or bad food for instance, are stored in the fat cells. If these are released into the system quickly during a spell of unaccustomed vigorous exercise and strict dieting, they are likely to make you feel quite ill. When you attend to the nutritional needs of your body by eating high-quality food, the body will require less to do the job in hand and your weight will normalise in time. It is quite unnecessary to pay a lot of money for fancy diets contained in tins and bottles. Never try to lose more than three pounds per week.

Most of us tend to think of fat being contained in butter, cheese, cream and meat. However, it is also present in eggs, nuts, whole milk, margarine, pastry, oils, crisps, chocolate and a host of 'snack foods'. Lean meat also contains fat, as do sausages. One very easy way to cut down on fat intake is by changing to skimmed milk rather than whole, and low-fat vegetable spreads instead of butter. If you find it difficult to tolerate skimmed milk, try semi-skimmed to start with and then progress to skimmed. Children should have whole or semi-skimmed milk rather than skimmed, because they are growing. Cottage cheese or Edam are lower in fat than hard or full-fat soft cheeses. Fried foods are obviously very high in fat content. Grill meats rather than roast or fry. If you are a chip fan, change to oven chips and avoid eating them more than once or (at the most) twice a week. Many dairy products and other foodstuffs are now labelled 'low-fat', so alternatives are easier to find.

In cold weather you will probably find that you crave more fatty foods than in warmer temperatures. This is one of the body's preservation techniques to insulate itself and maintain body heat. Many people find that their winter weight is three or four pounds over their summer weight and that the excess is shed easily once warmer weather commences.

Puddings are typically high in sugar and fat. Substitute fresh fruit or low-fat yoghurts. If you love puddings and find it difficult to cut them out, then you should try eating smaller portions of them, and then only on two or three days of the week. Remember that this will be more difficult if you have a sugar addiction.

● *Protein.*
An essential part of all our diets, especially for children, it is

used in growth and repair of the body's organs. It is contained in meat, soya, fish, milk, eggs, rice, cheese, beans, lentils, beanshoots, bread and certain vegetables and fruits. Some protein should be eaten at every meal. However, the British obsession with protein has caused the general diet to be top-heavy with these foods, creating an imbalance, with less importance placed on other vital ingredients in our diet such as fibre and vitamins.

The fact that meat has been highlighted as a major source of protein has led to our high consumption of animal produce. Vegetarians will vouch for the fact that it is perfectly possible to maintain a healthy (they would say healthier) lifestyle without meat. Red meat is a good source of iron and zinc as well as protein. However, it is possible to find iron in red lentils or leafy greens and zinc in fish or dried brewer's yeast. Unfortunately, many farmers find it necessary to pump their animals full of hormones and antibiotics to promote growth and improve yield. There is now a movement towards 'organic' meat farming where the animals are allowed a happy, if short, life without the use of artificial chemicals. Some butchers have realised the abhorrence many people feel at factory farming methods and at the use of chemicals which are being passed, via the food chain, into humans.

When you begin to eat a healthier diet, try cutting your red meat consumption down to two meals per week. Chicken and fish might be eaten on another two days, supplemented by three vegetarian days. Buy a good vegetarian cookery book so that the food is presented as a complete meal and your family are not searching around their plates for a piece of meat! Another good tip is to reduce the amount of mincemeat you use in bolognese sauce or shepherd's pie and make up the difference with red lentils.

● *Vitamins.*
The vitamin content of food is often destroyed during the preparation and cooking process. From the minute they are harvested fruit and vegetables begin to deteriorate, so it is essential that you eat them within a couple of days of buying

them. Milk left in daylight on the doorstep loses half its vitamin B2 (riboflavin) content within two hours. Cutting an orange in half or slicing green vegetables with a knife reduces the vitamin content. Soaking vegetables and boiling them to a soggy pulp will mean that most of the vitamins originally contained in them end up in the water which you throw down the sink!

Prepare vegetables just before cooking and then steam, pressure-cook or microwave them until they are tender but crisp. Whenever possible use raw fruit and vegetables in salads rather than cooked. Alternatively, cook them in a casserole or soup as you will then eat the liquid they have been cooked in along with the vegetables. Bake your potatoes rather than boiling or frying them. Eat the skins as well – they are rich in vitamins and a good source of fibre.

The vitamins in your body will be depleted by stress, pollution, smoking, drinking, drugs and the contraceptive pill. These factors make it more important for you to ensure that you do not destroy vitamins at their source, i.e. in your food intake. If you are susceptible to any of the above list of factors or are pregnant, then it is wise to take extra vitamins in tablet form. Children and elderly people should also take vitamin supplements to ensure that their supply is adequate. Vitamin tablets should always be taken after food in order to maximise their effects as they will be absorbed during digestion. Try to find a brand of vitamin tablet which does not contain preservatives.

● *Minerals.*

Along with vitamins, minerals play an important part in your body's functions. These are: calcium, iron, magnesium, phosphorus, sulphur, potassium, sodium, chloride, iodine and zinc. There is also a group of trace minerals which are important in nutritional value but required in minute doses. The same principles apply to these as to vitamins. Any overcooked or processed foods will be lacking in the correct minerals. Wholefoods will contain all the nutrients you require to maintain good health.

It is equally important not to overdose on vitamins and

minerals and so upset the delicate balance required for the healthy function of your whole system as it is to make sure you are getting enough. Unless you have reason to believe that you are deficient in a particular vitamin, then it is unnecessary for you to use a dietary supplement.

Always choose fresh food over prepared and packaged food. Never buy fruit or vegetables which have signs of ageing. If they are beginning to go off, there will be toxins contained in them which are likely to poison your system. Green potatoes are one of the worst examples and should never be eaten. Organically grown foods are best of all as they haven't been treated with chemical fertilisers or pesticides.

The next-best choice nutritionally after fresh fruit and vegetables are those you fresh-freeze yourself as you will know how old they are and that they do not contain preservatives. Cut down on your consumption of tinned and packaged foods which have been through lengthy processing before they reach you. Avoid keeping food in plastic film as it has been shown that carcinogenic substances are left in food which has been wrapped in plastic for any length of time. If you buy food wrapped this way, remove the film as soon as you get home. When using a microwave, ensure that plastic film used to cover dishes does not come into contact with the food during cooking.

Once again, good eating habits begin in the shops or supermarket. Plan your meals for the week in advance to ensure that they are balanced and varied. Make a list of the ingredients you require so that you are not tempted to buy the sort of processed, unhealthy products often seductively packaged and displayed. Some of the major supermarkets have now begun to label their products according to their nutritional value, making it easier for you to choose food wisely and health-consciously.

Healthy eating patterns

Now you have given some thought to *what* you eat, you can start to consider the *way* in which you eat. How many meals do you eat in a day? Are you continually eating snacks between meals or do you starve yourself all day only to binge all evening? Do you feel satisfied when you have eaten a meal or are you looking for more food within a short time of finishing?

Your lifestyle will have quite a significant effect on your eating habits. If you are a person who rises late, you are unlikely to sit and eat breakfast, being more inclined to have a piece of toast and a cup of coffee 'on the run'. This is likely to leave you feeling tired with reduced powers of concentration by mid-morning, probably craving sweets or a caffeine-loaded beverage. Do you sit down to eat a meal at lunchtime, or do you consider dinner in the evening to be your main meal of the day? Is your main meal eaten in front of the television whilst sitting in an armchair? Once again, examine your eating patterns and consider if they are a hindrance to your goal of achieving good health.

It is generally agreed among both medical and alternative practitioners that the best way of eating is exemplified in the old adage of 'Breakfast like a king, lunch like a prince and sup like a pauper.' Think of breakfast as a time of refuelling, with high-grade nourishment for the busy day ahead. A full stomach at night will prevent you from sleeping well and therefore from waking refreshed. Calories taken in late at night will not burn up during sleep, so that fat cells are more likely to be deposited. As a rule, do not eat after eight o'clock at night. Also, if you starve yourself during the day you will find yourself becoming increasingly nervy and more susceptible to the temptation of sweet food.

Take all your meals sitting at a table to ensure good posture which will aid your digestive process. Eat your food from a smaller plate so that the amounts seem larger. Present your food appetisingly with plenty of colourful garnish and side dishes. Chew your food thoroughly, taking time to experience the taste and texture of the food rather than bolting it quickly. Digestion begins in the mouth, and you will feel more satisfied at the end of a meal if you have spent time in the enjoyment of eating it. Never take any exercise or bathe immediately following a meal.

A good breakfast should contain fibre, protein, carbohydrate and vitamins. Ideally, on waking a glass of fruit juice or mineral water should be taken to cleanse the digestive system. Following a few exercises and a shower, solid nourishment in the form of a wholefood breakfast, containing bran, fruit, nuts and cereal, supplies all the required nutritional constituents. Muesli may be soaked in fruit juice overnight to soften it and make it more palatable. Alternatively, some fruit, natural 'live' yoghurt with a little wheatgerm and honey added, plus a piece of wholemeal toast, is an excellent starter. Porridge is a superb hot breakfast during cold weather, and is especially good for those people who are known to have coronary heart disease. Although a fry-up is full of protein it is also perilously high in saturated fat content and low in fibre, so don't breakfast on fried eggs and bacon.

The main meal of the day, whether taken in the middle of the day or in the early evening, should always include some fresh vegetables and an item which will supply protein for your body's needs. Grilled fish, two vegetables such as carrots and broccoli, and a baked potato constitutes a perfectly balanced meal. Brown rice risottos, or wholewheat pasta such as a vegetable lasagne, are very filling and are nutritious meals which can be enjoyed by all the family.

The third, lighter meal may be a wholemeal sandwich, a salad (remember that salads can be far more interesting than a piece of lettuce and a tomato!), sugar-free beans on toast, or a jacket potato with extra filling. Fresh, homemade soups are particularly nourishing and can be eaten as either a main meal with warm wholemeal rolls or as a light snack. Keep the stock after boiling vegetables to make up soups with other vegetables and pulses.

Kitchen hygiene

Dirty cooking pots, cutlery, plates and work surfaces all encourage bacteria to multiply, so engendering diseases of the alimentary tract. These may range from a simple mouth ulcer to the dangerous salmonella infection. A badly cleaned milk pan is the perfect medium for bacteria to breed in. If this happens, the next occasion the pan is used the bacteria will contaminate the fresh food being cooked. Germs will also fester in the crevices of cracked crockery as these cannot be properly cleaned.

All utensils should be washed in very hot water and rinsed of all traces of detergent in clean cool water. If possible they should then be left to drain and dry in their own time rather than being rubbed with a tea towel which may contain traces of food from when it was last used.

Work surfaces should be regularly scoured with hot water to remove any traces of food. If you are preparing chicken, *never* place it on a wooden surface, as this will retain any salmonella bacteria present even after washing. Only bleach will remove these bacteria from the wood.

In olden days most people cooked their food in large iron cooking pots which actually helped them to maintain the iron levels in their blood. This was due to the fact that minute particles of the pots came off into the food and were ingested! These days our cookware is more likely to be made of aluminium or enamelled metal or coated with non-stick chemical compounds. These may actually be highly toxic when used over a long period of time for preparing food. Some coloured enamelled pans contain lead and cadmium which are highly toxic. Severe metal poisoning can cause appalling symptoms associated with brain deterioration and is particularly dangerous to children. The best pots are of non-enamelled iron or earthenware.

Germs will also breed in the sink, drain, dishmop and in cutlery holders, so these require regular cleaning. The tin-opener is another oft-forgotten utensil when it comes to being washed up. These small points are all important when it comes to maintaining kitchen hygiene.

4
Physical fitness

Every morning the Japanese nation bend, stretch, balance and move their way through a set of disciplined exercises designed to help them make a healthy start to the day, in the belief that a fit workforce will enable high productivity in the factories.

The benefits of regular exercise are now well-publicised. Recent years have shown the leisure industry to be a major growth area, providing facilities for all members of the community and, encouraging us to take up a sport or exercise class both for enjoyment and to improve fitness. Those who experience the beneficial results of regular physical exercise often become 'hooked' on it and will testify to the positive effects on their whole welfare. Many people, especially women, take up exercise for the aesthetic value and some because of medical advice, particularly heart patients. Whatever the reason for the initial movement towards regular exercise, it is important to choose a form suited to your individual personality type and within your own physical capabilities.

Although exercise is important for your physical well-being, it is really only a part of the picture. The exhilaration felt after a swim or a long walk is excellent for the morale and for improving your mental outlook. The level of concentration required for most types of exercise relieves the mind of its other worries for a time. The self-discipline needed to follow a set of movements in order to improve your performance in a chosen sport can be very satisfying. There is also the added benefit of meeting people who have chosen to take up the same activity as you. All of these aspects of exercise send positive and healthy messages to your mind, body and spirit.

Muscles require a good oxygen supply to function correctly,

as do all the organs of the body. The supply of oxygen is increased during physical exertion, causing the blood to circulate faster, carrying that essential supply around the body and removing waste so that it can be excreted via the kidneys. Exercise, therefore, has the added benefit of cleansing the system, ridding your body of waste products which have built up from daily living. A sluggish system which does not receive these benefits becomes stagnant and toxic, leading to lethargy and perhaps eventually to illness. It is important when embarking upon a regular exercise routine to build up the amount of exertion gradually so that accumulated toxins are not released too quickly into the system or in too large amounts.

Building up your exercise routine slowly also makes sense for the more obvious reasons of muscle strain and injury. Our muscles are designed to hold the skeleton and organs of the body in place, as well as to facilitate a full range of movements. For them to be able to do this job adequately they require tone, and if they become flabby or wasted through not being used properly then they cannot carry out this important function. To keep their correct tone, it is essential to exercise the muscles. However, overworking the muscles through continual tension, overstretching or too much exercise can lead to aching and injury and prevent the free flow of blood around the system, causing a lack of oxygen which is detrimental to other parts of the body.

In order for exercise to be totally effective it should be balanced with correct posture, breathing and relaxation so that the benefits gained from activity are maintained and built upon. This chapter is designed to help you build a regime incorporating all of these, enabling you to feel fitter.

Breathing

The phrase 'natural as breathing' indicates that this is an activity we carry out without having to think about it. That is, unless something interferes to make it uncomfortable or difficult. Part of the brain is designed to control automatically our breathing rate, heart rate and all other bodily functions over which seemingly we have very little conscious control. Because of this subconscious action, breathing is often neglected as part of a health programme. When you breathe in, carbon dioxide, the waste product in the blood, is exchanged for oxygen via the lungs. Freshly oxygenated blood is then pumped around the body by the heart and the carbon dioxide is breathed out.

Movement is essential to the healthy functioning of the lungs and other breathing apparatus. It is for this reason that immobile patients must have physiotherapy so that the lungs can be cleared of the mucus which collects around the breathing tubes that is usually moved naturally by physical activity. Pneumonia may eventually result if this mucus is not cleared. This is a particular hazard to the elderly who frequently develop this disease, especially if they are invalided and immobile.

All breathing should be done through the nose, both the breath in and the breath out. The mouth is primarily for the purpose for eating and should act in breathing only as a safety valve in case the nose becomes blocked. We do not use the full capacity of our lungs all the time and so there is always some lung power 'in reserve' for when we require extra oxygen, such as when we become afraid or need to exert ourselves physically. Both these things will use up energy and cause different muscle groups to work harder, requiring a larger supply of oxygen and so causing the breathing rate to increase into panting. However these unused parts of the lungs should be exercised deliberately each day in order to rid ourselves of the stagnant air which collects at the bottom of the lungs and also to oxygenate the blood fully. Known as aerobic, this type of exercise will keep all the breathing apparatus and its essential muscles in trim should it be required to work harder.

To increase your awareness of what happens when you breathe, try the following exercises.

- Place your hand in front of your face with the palm under your nose. Close your eyes and breathe in through your nose, all the time being aware of the cool air entering your body. As you breathe out notice how the breath takes a different route down your nose! The air is now moist and warm on your palm.

- Place the palms of your hands on your chest with the fingertips resting lightly on the collarbones. Take a normal breath in and out. You will notice that your chest moves up and out. Now move one hand to rest lightly over your abdomen where your ribs part into an inverted V-shape, leaving the other hand on your chest.

  When you breathe in this time, try to move the hand on your abdomen outwards without moving the upper chest. This action, known as 'diaphragmatic breathing', releases tension in the stomach muscles. When practised regularly this can be a marvellous aid to relaxation.

  Now move both hands to rest lightly on the sides of your ribs, just above your waist. On breathing in, try to move the ribs out to the sides keeping the upper chest still and without raising the stomach. These muscles and the lower part of the lungs are usually the least used.

- To take a full breath, start by raising the stomach as you breathe in, take the same breath into the sides and finish by filling out the upper chest! Breathe out! Aim to make the breath in last to a slow count of 10, by building up gradually, and make the breath out last the same amount of time.

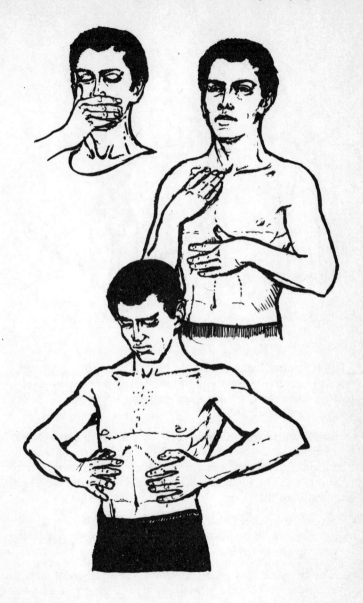

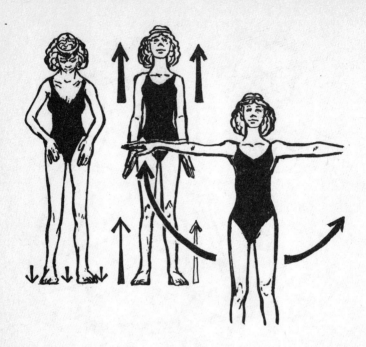

The following exercise should be practised in the morning and will help to oxygenate your blood fully for the day ahead, clearing your mind of sleep and revving up your circulatory system for the day ahead.

- Stand with the feet shoulder-width apart, weight evenly distributed under each foot. Ensure that the tailbone is tucked in and that the shoulders are relaxed rather than hunched. The head should be straight with the chin held parallel to the floor.

- Stretch the whole body upwards as though a cord were attached to the centre of the scalp pulling towards the ceiling! Do not raise your heels from the floor.

- Slowly raise both arms sideways until they are at shoulder level, taking a deep breath in (through your nose) as you do so.

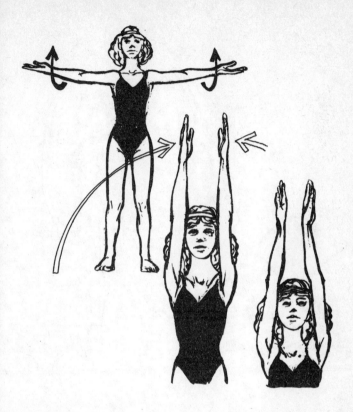

- Rotate the arms outwards until both palms are facing the ceiling, breathing out (through your nose) as you turn them.

- Now take your arms upwards again until your fingers are pointing to the ceiling and your inner arms are next to your ears, breathing in as you do this.

- Hold this breath for a slow count of five and turn your palms to face away from your body. Ensure you keep the upward stretch on your whole body and the weight even under both feet, making certain your heels are still on the floor.

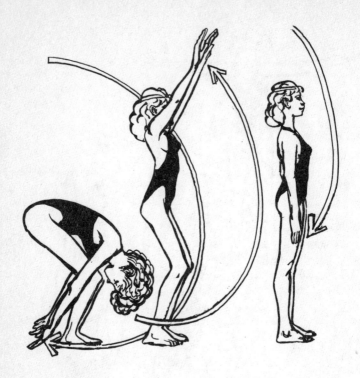

- Now sweep downwards to the floor, bending both knees, taking the arms straight to the floor and backwards behind you, breathing out as you do so.

- As you uncurl to stand up again, bring both arms up in front of you until they are pointing towards the ceiling again, taking a breath in as you come up. Make sure you bend your knees and take your weight in your legs and thighs as you up come so that stress is not put on your lower back.

- Slowly lower arms to your sides, breathing out slowly.

Repeat five times gradually building up to 10.

When you practise this, add a little bounce as you sweep down to the floor and take your arms behind you. Keep all the movements fluid and smooth rather than jerking. Carry out the exercise in a room which has fresh air in it – there is no point to the exertion if you do it in a bedroom which has stale air from the night before! Use it to help you if you find yourself nodding off in the office, and remember to open a window first.

Posture

There is perhaps no easier way of correctly establishing a person's frame of mind than by observing the way he or she is holding him- or herself in either a sitting or standing posture. The way we feel about ourselves, the rest of the world and the manner in which we live are all apparent in our physical stance. Note the round-shouldered, bent posture of people said to have the 'cares of the world on their shoulders'. Modern furniture, shoes and methods of transport add to the problems. As we live all of our lives being pulled down by the effects of gravity, it seems easier to succumb to slumping forwards.

Poor posture actually uses excess energy, as muscles are tensed unnecessarily in the wrong alignment, putting undue stress on them and eventually leading to fatigue. Free blood flow becomes restricted by the muscle tension, causing stagnation in certain areas, and the internal organs are squashed so that there is inadequate room for their healthy function. The whole system suffers if posture is incorrect, but perhaps the most common problems are those related to the spine and the resulting back difficulties.

Poor posture usually begins early in life, around the time when children start school and begin to slouch over their desks. If you decide to make the effort to improve your posture, not only will the effects be obvious in your general health but the difference in the way other people react to you will also be apparent. There is no doubt that we react more positively to those who hold themselves upright, thereby appearing more self-possessed, confident and positive in their outlook. (Do not rely upon good posture only, however, in order to build your self-confidence. That can only really come from within.)

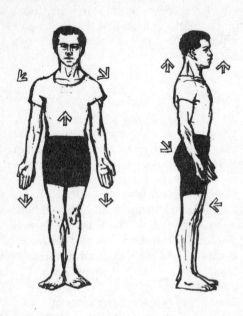

● *Standing.* A truly correct standing posture is relaxed, balanced and erect. Unfortunately, when people are asked to 'stand up straight' they tend to hunch their shoulders, throw out their chest and stick their chin in the air – highly uncomfortable!

Practise correct standing by following these steps. It sounds a lot of trouble but comes naturally after a while. Standing in front of a mirror helps to correct the faults.

● Stand with the feet together, matching toe joints, ankle bones and inner knees. Rock your weight back slightly on to the heels and spread the toes evenly, then place the weight fully on to the whole foot. The instep should be the only part to be clear of the floor. This will give you a firm base on which to balance.

● Pull up through the legs, keeping the knees together and pushing the front thighs back. This may have the effect of tilting the pelvis backwards so in order to counteract this, push the base of the spine towards the floor. (If your bottom is sticking out, tuck it in!).

● Lift the whole ribcage (front and back) upwards. The shoulders should stretch downwards and out to the sides. Stretch the hands towards the floor and then relax them. The inside of the arms should face forwards.

● Stretch the neck and head upwards without tilting the chin.

Throughout this exercise, try to feel taller and keep a mental image of 'growing' in your mind. Your weight should be kept evenly balanced under both feet.

● *Sitting.* All the rules which apply to standing also apply to a good basic sitting position. That is, the weight should be distributed evenly throughout the body with both feet placed flat on the ground.

● As you seat yourself, ensure that you place the haunch bones on the chair rather than the tailbone or base of your spine. Your back should rest lightly against the back of the chair.

● Place the feet evenly and slightly apart on the floor.

● Stretch the spine upwards and the shoulders downwards and out to the sides. Rest the hands gently on your lap, palms upwards, allowing the fingers to curl naturally. Make sure you do not feel tense around your shoulders.

Research has shown that in order to hold the spine truly erect when sitting, the thighs should slope downwards and the knees bend backwards at 45°. Small children naturally sit this way when they are playing on the floor and chairs have now been designed to help achieve this posture. As this obviously involves some expense, a similar effect can be gained by raising the back legs of an upright chair so that the seat slopes downwards. Crossing your legs causes poor circulation eventually leading to varicose veins.

A good seated posture is particularly important whilst you are eating so that the gullet, stomach and other digestive organs have room to function properly.

● *Active posture.* Good posture does not just apply to standing or sitting still. Once you have mastered the basic technique of holding a relaxed, balanced and upright position, then the rules can also be applied to walking, dancing, driving, lifting and all daily activities. With practice it will become a habit.

● *Lifting.* One of the most common reasons for loss of working days is back problems. Spinal ailments are not only extremely painful but also cause a feeling of general ill-health. This is due to the fact that all the nerves of the body are linked to the spinal cord which is encircled by the vertebral bones of the spine. The majority of minor back injuries are caused by incorrectly lifting heavy objects, wrongly taking the weight in the muscles of the back rather than in those of the legs.

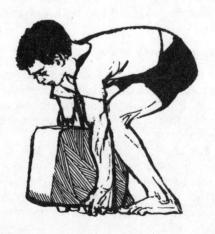

● *Driving.* If you drive for a living then it is doubly important to adopt the correct position so that tensions are not wrongly created, leading to stiffness in the muscles and, therefore, to excessive tiredness. The mental concentration required for driving is quite tiring enough without the added drain on energy reserves from improper muscle use!

Ensure that when you seat yourself in your vehicle you are centred in the middle of the driving seat with your bottom against the back. The back of the seat should be in an upright position and your feet should touch the pedals without having to stretch your legs or bend up your knees uncomfortably. Your arms should be slightly bent at the elbows and should reach the steering wheel straight out in front of you, so that you are not having to twist to either side. When holding the steering wheel, a gentle pressure is preferable to a tight grip which causes all the arm and shoulder muscles to work twice as hard as is really necessary. Keep your back against the seat and avoid hunching your shoulders or slouching over the wheel.

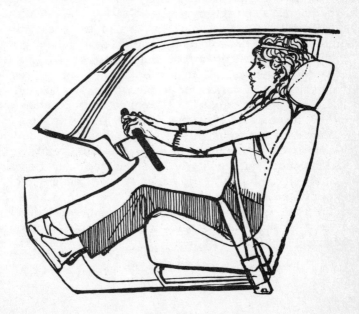

Although you are now aware of the reasons why exercise plays such an important part in a total health programme, actually choosing the sort of activity suitable for you and then sticking to it is a different matter altogether. If you have led a very sedentary lifestyle thus far and have decided to begin exercising regularly, it would not be advisable initially to take up an extremely rigorous sport such as squash, as the shock to your system may be too great and so cause damage. In order for exercise to be beneficial it should be hard enough to raise your heartbeat (and a sweat) without causing the sort of breathlessness which precludes conversation!

Regular, small amounts of exercise are far more beneficial than large doses once a month. It is better to start by spending 10 minutes three days a week on your chosen activity, gradually building up to an hour on three days, or more if you feel like it. If you decide to take up swimming, for instance, you would start by swimming one or two lengths the first week, four the second week, six on the third week and so on. Once you are feeling fitter you may decide to take up another complementary activity in order to develop different skills and sets of muscles.

The following table shows groups of exercises graded according to the fitness requirement. Those in the first group are particularly useful for basic fitness and are beneficial for improving abilities in other sports. They are especially recommended as starters for people whose greatest exertion is pressing the button on the TV remote control, as they can all be tailored to individual ability. These activities, if practised as recommended, will not throw any sudden, violent stress on the heart or other muscles. Group two is recommended for people who feel they are already basically fit and can comfortably carry out an activity from group one. Group three is reserved for those who are young (under 35) and very fit. Group four contains those sports which develop specialised skills and strengths in particular muscle groups and require good basic fitness.

EXERCISE TABLE

ONE	TWO	THREE	FOUR
Walking	Golf	Aerobic dancing	Windsurfing
Swimming	Tennis	Squash	Ice skating
Cycling	Badminton	Weight-lifting	Horse riding
Jogging	Keep-fit	Competitive racing (any sport)	Yachting
Yoga		Athletics	

Daily exercise plan

If you feel you haven't the time or inclination to take up a sport, 10–15 minutes of exercise per day is all that is required to keep you basically fit. The following exercise plan is designed to keep firm muscle tone, speed up the circulatory system and exercise the heart and lungs. Whenever you exercise it is important to warm the muscles up slowly so that they can stretch easily in order to avoid injury.

- Stand straight and tall using the guide on page 60. Keep stretching the whole body in this way for 30 seconds.

- Remain standing straight. Rotate alternate shoulders backwards five times each. Circle both shoulders together five times.

- Lightly jog and shake both hands loosely from the wrists at the same time for one minute.

- Practise the breathing exercise described on page 56 five times.

- Stand with your feet apart. Bend sideways from the waist, making sure you do not twist your spine. Push your fingertips down your thigh, going down only as far as is comfortable within your own stretching range.

- Lie flat on the floor. Lift one leg about 12–18 inches from

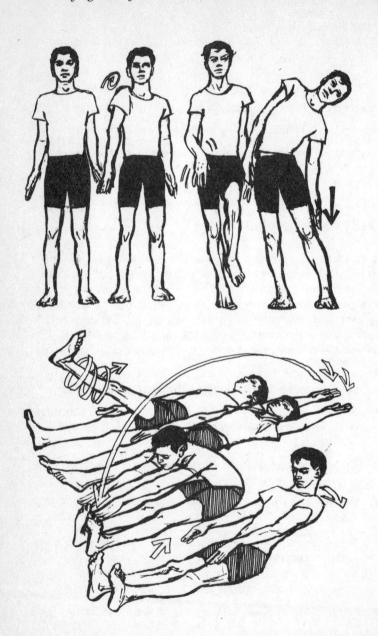

the floor and rotate the foot five times in a clockwise direction and then anticlockwise another five times. Repeat with the other leg.

- Stay on the floor and take your hands over your head, placing them behind you on the floor. Stretch your whole body from fingertips to toes. Raise yourself to a sitting position while bringing your arms over your head and stretch forward to touch your toes. Gently lower the top half of your body back to the floor using your stomach muscles (not your arms) and stretch your arms above your head once more. Repeat five times. If your stomach muscles are weak or if you have any back problems, hook your toes under a solid piece of furniture and bend your knees up.

- Finish by repeating the first, stretching exercise.

As your fitness improves you will be able to increase the number of times you do each exercise within the time available. The exercise routine we have suggested is a very gentle one which most people could start practising immediately, but if you know you are very unfit or have special health problems, check with your doctor before beginning any exercise programme.

We would suggest that morning is the best time of day to practise these exercises, but do not jump out of bed and immediately start exercising. Have a drink and read the paper first, allowing yourself time to wake up! Always exercise before eating, never just after. If you have eaten a meal then allow at least an hour before starting to exercise in order to allow the digestive process to work properly. This applies particularly to swimming.

One final word of warning. If you have been ill with a viral or bacterial infection, wait until you are completely recovered before you start exercising again. Muscles become weakened during illness and if you place any undue strain on them too soon it could be dangerous. This is especially relevant to the heart, as it is mainly made up of muscle tissue. Never throw yourself back into strenuous exercise after any illness or long break and always build up gradually in order to avoid injury.

Sports injuries

If you are unfortunate enough to injure yourself while participating in a sporting activity, first aid treatment is very important. Soft issue injuries involve muscles, ligaments or tendons, which can be torn, strained or bruised. When treating these injuries the word to remember is ICE. This stands for Ice, Compression and Elevation. The sooner this is carried out after the injury the quicker it is likely to heal. Press ice over the affected part (a bag of frozen peas is ideal!). Apply firm, even pressure to the injury over the ice. If possible elevate the injured limb.

Serious injury such as suspected broken bones should obviously be seen by a medical practitioner immediately. However, if it is less serious but does not seem to be healing with rest, then a medical opinion should be sought within a few days. Specialised sports injury clinics are now becoming more common and are usually privately run. Never restart your sport until the injury is healed and until it has been tested less strenuously.

In order to avoid these types of injuries there are a set of very simple rules to be followed. These are:

- Always warm up slowly before vigorous exercise by stretching, bending and jogging. This is especially important in cold weather. A cold muscle is far less elastic than a warm one.

- Never overstretch your limits. It is necessary to push yourself a little further each time you exercise in order to improve, but progress must be gradual.

- If you have a weak muscle do not put unnecessary strain on it.

Relaxation

True relaxation of mind and body is not easy to achieve but is essential to good health. It has to be practised regularly in order to free all the tensions which have collected over the day. Sleep is not equal to complete relaxation as our brains are still busy and we continue to move around. Many people find deep relaxation difficult to achieve as it is something which we have to 'allow' to happen rather than actively 'do'. Once it is mastered, however, it can be an invaluable aid to good health, relieving stress within a few minutes.

As you are learning to relax, choose a soothing piece of music which you can associate with your period of relaxation. Each time you practise, listen to this particular tune so that when you hear it you will immediately start to 'let go'. A darkened room is preferable to bright light, especially to rest your eyes. Find a comfortable position which allows you to have the least tension in your muscles. This may be sitting or lying, but ensure that you feel balanced and unrestricted. For instance, do not curl up to one side, and ensure that your limbs are not crossed and that you are not wearing any tight clothing.

When you feel comfortable close your eyes. Mentally say to yourself that nothing matters at this moment – and believe it! Starting at your toes, work your way up through your whole body ensuring that each part is free of tension. If a particular muscle does not feel relaxed, actively tense and release it until it feels loose. The muscles of the stomach, hands, neck, shoulders and face are particularly prone to stress and should be checked several times to ensure they are completely at ease. Your jaw should not be clenched and your tongue should lie loosely on the floor of your mouth.

When you feel that your muscles are without tension, bring your concentration to your breathing. Using the 'diaphragmatic breath' described on page 54, slowly breathe in to a count of 10. Hold the breath for 5 to 10 seconds and then slowly breathe out (through your nose!), again for a count of 10. When you have done this a few times and are feeling quieter, allow your breathing to become shallow, slow and even.

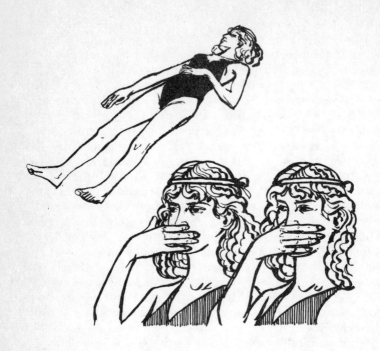

Now concentrate on allowing your body to feel heavier, sinking down into the bed or whatever you are resting on. Your aim is to reach a deeper, more tranquil level of consciousness, not to fall asleep. You should still be aware of what is going on around you. However, if you are having difficulty falling asleep at night, this type of breathing can be used to induce sleep. If you are feeling particularly over-wrought and find it difficult to empty your mind of thought, try humming on one note as you breathe out through your nose. Alternatively, try slowly repeating a monosyllabic word, such as 'one' or 'hum', over and over to yourself until you feel calmer. You will eventually find that you can relax easily, switching off your train of thought for a few minutes and subsequently feeling more refreshed.

When you are unable to lie down in order to relax, this yoga exercise can be extremely beneficial for inducing relaxation. Lightly squeeze your nose between your thumb and forefinger so that both nostrils are closed. Your mouth should remain shut. Remove your thumb and breathe in through the open nostril. Replace your thumb and remove your forefinger and breathe out. Repeat this a couple of times and then change over so that you breathe in through the other side of your nose in order to achieve a balance.

Visualisation

Once you become proficient at the art of deep relaxation, you will be able to use it to improve different aspects of your health which you feel need attention by incorporating visualisation. When your body is totally at rest and your mind is completely quiet, use your imagination to create healing images for that part of your body which is sick, or in order to increase your energy levels. This technique is now quite commonly used as part of the therapy to help cancer patients. For instance if you have a headache or stomach upset, imagine the affected area being flooded with a bright, healing energy. Keep this image in your head for several minutes at a time. As you practise this, try to allow it to feel as real as possible. You may actually experience a tingling feeling in the area you are concentrating on. The more real you feel it, the more benefit you will gain.

To increase your energy levels, imagine a small, bright, throbbing ball of light, representing pure energy, centred just above your navel. Allow this to grow and spread, bathing all your body in a refreshing glow so that you tingle from head to toe. You will need to be quite well-practised at deep relaxation before you find this very beneficial.

When you are ending your period of relaxation, move slowly rather than jumping up and immediately exerting yourself once again. Quicken your breathing slightly and stretch your limbs. If you are lying on your back, roll on to your side. Finally, open your eyes.

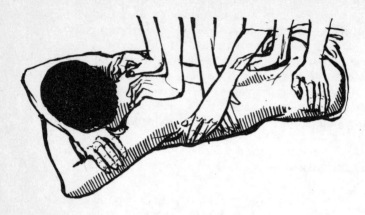

Massage

As aids to relaxation go, there can be few more sensual experiences than massage. It can also be used to improve the circulation, ease muscle aches and as a technique to improve specific ailments. For complementary practitioners such as osteopaths, chiropractors, acupressurists and reflexologists, massage is a vital part of therapy. The use of massage as an aid to healing is very ancient. We are urged as small children to 'rub it better' if we should hurt ourselves, and often apply this rule to emotional hurt also. Our gut response to another person who is upset is often to hug or stroke them.

In order to give a really good massage, the strokes should be firm but gentle. Oil or lotion should be used to reduce the friction on the skin and the finishing stroke should always be towards the heart.

This is a way to massage the muscles of the back and is superbly relaxing. The person being massaged should lie flat on his or her stomach with arms folded under their head. Ensure that he or she is warm enough.

As masseur or masseuse place your hands, palms down, either side of the spine just above the buttocks. Apply even pressure through the thumbs using wide, circular motions working your way up the back. When you reach the shoulder and neck area, knead the flesh between your fingers and thumbs as this is an area which gathers much tension. Now work your way back down the sides one at a time by stroking the flesh under the armpit in the direction of the spine, crossing one hand over the other in a fluid motion.

If you are not lucky enough to have someone who will provide a massage for you, there are a number of massage aids which can be bought so that you can give yourself a massage. These range from rubber mitts for use in the shower to little wooden ducks or fish on wheels! For tired feet, try rolling a tennis ball around under the soles of your feet, while walking on sand or shale in the sea is a great boost for the whole system.

Sleep

The amount of sleep you require will depend upon the many factors which apply to you as an individual. Children require more sleep than adults and the elderly. Some people can manage with only 3 or 4 hours in 24 whereas others require a full 10. American researchers found in their experiments that the people who had less sleep were more energetic and lively than those who took 8 to 10 hours per night, who seemed to be more lethargic. It seems that quality of sleep is more important than the actual quantity.

For sleep to be truly beneficial, both the mind and body need to be peaceful. One of the most obvious signs of depression is awakening in the early hours of the morning and ruminating over one's worries. A large meal and stimulants such as caffeine or alcohol can have a detrimental effect on the quality of your sleep. Sleep-inducing drugs, known as hypnotics, can never replace the body's own hormones in producing restful sleep. The brain patterns of those patients who take them are quite different from those of people who do not. These drugs are also frequently addictive, so that a person who has been taking them for a long time cannot rest without their aid. They should always be used with the utmost caution. Insomnia can be due to calcium deficiency. This is possibly why the milky drink is popular at bedtime, as it has a high calcium content. Nervousness can also be due to a lack of vitamin B which is contained in wholegrain cereals. Valerian and camomile are two herbal remedies for insomnia.

During sleep, your body's metabolism slows down and vital repair work to the cells is carried out. Dreams are an important part of the sleep pattern. Troubled dreams are often a sign of mental or emotional anguish and, as such, should not be ignored. They can be used to help you get to the root of disturbed feelings. Many psychotherapists ask their clients to keep a 'dream diary' recording their dreams in as much detail as they can remember. These are later examined during therapy.

Stress, with its resulting tension, is one of the main causative factors of serious disease. It is not possible to live life without some turmoil, but you can learn to cope with it without stress and learn how to lessen the side-effects, so reducing the chances of it ruining your health in the long term.

5
Stages of life

As one generation gives birth to the next, so life's cycle continues. Although each person is unique, we share our humanity. Each of us is conceived, born and eventually dies. The cycle may be long or tragically short, but in between birth and death are several lifestages to be managed. All of us will experience at least one or more of these critical stages.

Throughout life, change is inevitable, though often resisted. Coming to terms with the changes taking place enables growth of the personality, and is an enriching experience which you can draw upon when confronted with a new situation. Slow changes such as adolescence and ageing, as well as the more dramatic such as birth and death, can create the life crises. How you as an individual cope will depend very much on your own personality and view of life.

We tend to think of life as beginning at birth and ending with death, but in fact the nine months spent in the womb are some of the most important and dramatic in terms of change, growth and development that any of us will ever experience. For this reason, we have begun our lifestages chapter at preconception, when a being is thought about even before actually existing.

PRE-PREGNANCY

In a perfect world all the babies born would be planned, wanted and loved. They would be raised by two loving parents, nurtured and cared for until old enough to take care of themselves. Unless you are living in Cloud-cuckoo-land, you will know that this, of course, is not the case. The majority of the world's children are probably unplanned. Starting out as a mistake is not the best way to begin life. Even those children referred to as 'happy accidents' can feel insecure about their presence in the family. Feelings of resentment on the part of the parents are often hard to disguise, no matter how deep the parents try to bury them.

In the 1950s and 1960s it was quite common for couples experiencing matrimonial difficulties to be advised to have another baby in order to cement the marriage together. With hindsight we can see that, in many cases, all this did was to produce another blameless person who had to suffer emotional trauma as the child of a broken marriage. The pressures of pregnancy, childbirth and coping with a new baby are difficult enough for a couple with a stable relationship to bear, let alone those having problems. Parenthood can be one of life's most rewarding experiences, but make sure that it happens only when *you* want it to.

Emotional issues apart, there are many physical aspects affecting the unborn child which need to be looked at before a pregnancy begins. If, as a woman, you are taking any drugs then your system will need time to clean these out before you start a pregnancy. The contraceptive pill should be stopped three months before even trying to conceive as it depletes the vitamin supply of the body as well as affecting hormone balance. Check whether you have had German measles or have been vaccinated against it as a girl. Do not hesitate to ask your doctor about this as it is one risk that is totally unnecessary. Should you catch German measles in the early stages of pregnancy, your baby will have a high chance of being born seriously handicapped. If you do get vaccinated as an adult it is extremely important to allow at least three months, using barrier contraception, before attempting to conceive.

Should you have a condition such as epilepsy which is controlled by drugs and are unable to stop taking them, always check with your doctor as to whether it is safe to attempt a pregnancy on the usual dosage. Heart patients and those women suffering from kidney problems should also discuss with their doctor in advance the effects of pregnancy on their health. Obesity is an added risk to pregnant women, due to the extra strain put on the heart and also because the obese tend to have high blood pressure which can risk the lives of both mother and baby. A healthy low-fat, high-fibre diet with very little salt, sugar or food additives should be followed during the months when you are attempting to conceive and throughout pregnancy (see Chapter 3).

It is imperative to stop smoking before you become pregnant rather than when you have a pregnancy confirmed. If your partner or work colleagues smoke you should also encourage them to give up so that you are not inhaling their fumes. There is conclusive evidence that the babies of couples who smoke are born underweight. This is particularly critical if the child is born prematurely. Every time you inhale cigarette smoke your baby is deprived of some of its vital oxygen supply. Parenting involves a lot of unselfishness, and it begins here!

Alcohol and drug abuse also present dangers to the foetus and can result in deformity. Some babies of drug addicts are also addicted and suffer withdrawal symptoms within a few days of being born. There have been cases where mothers of these babies have been convicted of abusing their unborn children. Although the ethics of this are questionable, it does bring very forcibly to our attention the presence of a new person before its emergence into the world.

It is for this reason that X-rays and ultraviolet sunbeds should also be strictly avoided around the time you are attempting to conceive. Although no conclusive evidence has been found for UV beds causing deformity of newborn infants, no one is absolutely sure that they are innocent either. Radiation from X-rays is known positively to cause problems during the early part of pregnancy. You will not be sure you are pregnant until the foetus is two and possibly three weeks old, when the cell division is most rapid and development crucial. If you have the least suspicion that you might be pregnant, avoid coming into contact with substances known to affect an unborn child. These include certain chemicals. If you work in the chemical industry, check with your employer as to whether you should be moved when you start trying to conceive.

For a pregnancy to occur, a sperm from the male partner must meet up with and fertilise the egg or ovum in the female. An egg is usually released each month, about 14 days after the first day of the last period. This egg lives for about three days and, if it is not fertilised, is shed with the lining of the womb in the next period. This means that each woman is usually only capable of becoming pregnant for about three or four days in each menstrual cycle. If sexual intercourse does not occur during this fertile time then a pregnancy cannot occur.

If you are actively trying to conceive, it is therefore quite useful to know when ovulation occurs. Some women know instinctively when this is. They have certain body changes such as increased, clear vaginal secretions and in some instances even an increase in sexual desire. It is possible to pinpoint the fertile period using a temperature chart or chemical kit which detects hormonal changes in the urine.

Women's age does make a difference to their ability to conceive. Once over 30, fertility starts to decline and so becoming pregnant can take longer than for a younger woman. Women who are very anxious to become pregnant often experience difficulty in conceiving. This would seem to be linked to stress and may be a natural defence reflex for both the mother and the not-yet-conceived child. It is very often the case that when no reason can be found for infertility occurring, the couple eventually adopt and then conceive their own child quite quickly afterwards!

PREGNANCY

If your period is late and you are sexually active, always consider pregnancy as the prime cause until it is proven otherwise. Tests have been known to be wrong. The home testing kits available now are usually sensitive enough to detect a pregnancy as early as the first day of the missed period. These kits work by detecting a hormone only present during pregnancy and excreted in the urine. However, if this test is negative and your period still does not arrive, you should repeat it after seven days. Most tests will give a positive result by this time if you are pregnant. By eight weeks, the time of the second missed period, a pregnancy is usually detectable by other signs and symptoms. The commonest of these are breast soreness, lethargy, nausea and having to pass water frequently.

Pregnancy is a highly emotive subject for those personally involved. Each woman wants the best care available and has different needs to be catered for. The tests carried out throughout the nine months are essential preventive measures for the continuance of a healthy pregnancy. Unfortunately, many women feel they have been 'taken over' as objects to be poked, prodded and pushed around. Antenatal clinics have been described as 'cattle markets', with good cause in some cases. Remember that you have a choice as to where you go to have your obstetric care. You may go to your own GP (if he or she is on the obstetric list), a hospital maternity clinic, or have shared care between your own doctor and the hospital consultant. If you are not happy with the hospital to which you have been referred, you should ask to be referred elsewhere. The main key to successful obstetric care is to ask questions whenever you do not understand what is happening and why. This will enable you to remain in control of the decisions made about your state of health.

Throughout your pregnancy you will be seen at regular intervals by midwives and obstetrically qualified doctors who monitor your progress and that of your unborn baby. This should begin as early as eight weeks into your pregnancy in order that any abnormalities can be found and dealt with appropriately.

Between 8 and 28 weeks your visits to the clinic should be every four weeks unless there is a specific problem, such as high blood pressure or anaemia, which requires treatment. Towards the end of the pregnancy, monitoring is more frequent and the visits increase to one each fortnight between 28 and 36 weeks. During the final month you are asked to attend each week. The detailed care of health through pregnancy and childbirth requires more space than is available here. There are many good books on the subject (see the Reading List on page 138). You should make sure you are well informed.

THE NEW-BORN BABY

For the first few weeks after birth mother and child are, paradoxically, going through a period of both separation and bonding. Seeing your child for the first time is an experience not unlike meeting someone whom you have only previously spoken to on the telephone! You feel as though you know them well but they don't look a bit like you think they should!

For the new mother there is the job of learning to feed her child and the horror of even considering she will have to pass another bowel movement – ever! (A mother's body can feel rather battered and sore after giving birth.) Although it is now a cliche, there is no doubt that breast *is* best. You will never have to worry about whether the milk formula is too strong or too weak, your baby will not get an infection from badly sterilised bottles and teats, you will not have to spend half the day making up bottles, and your baby will receive immunity to many diseases and will be less likely to die a cot death. Unfortunately, breastfeeding comes naturally to very few mothers. It is especially difficult for women with fair skins and flat nipples. However, with the right information and help it is possible to surmount the problems. There are several important rules to follow for successful breastfeeding. (For convenience's sake only we have referred to the baby and later the child as 'he' throughout.)

- Try to stay relaxed. If you you are tense your milk will not flow freely and this will lead to a vicious circle of hungry baby, tense mother, no milk and an even hungrier, frustrated and angry baby.

- Drink plenty of fluids. Mineral water and stout (in moderation) are excellent. Fruit juice can sometimes upset babies' tummies and should be drunk in small amounts only.

- Feed your baby on demand. If he is crying and you are certain he cannot possibly be hungry then he may just need to suck.

- If your supply seems to be diminished try drinking more fluids, stay relaxed, feed him more often and have plenty of rest.

- Ignore anyone who tries to put you off or discourage you. Have faith!

- When you have to feed your baby, ensure that you are not trying to do another job or hold a conversation at the same time. He needs *all* your attention.

- Never allow anyone to tell you that your supply is insufficient for a large baby. Twins can be successfully breastfed by one mother. Some mothers feed their baby entirely from one breast!

- If you become engorged and sore, express a *little* milk as soon as you feel full. Placing warm flannels over your breasts will help to release the flow.

- Should an abcess develop in one breast, feed normally from the other and take an appropriate antibiotic until it clears. Express the milk from the infected breast and throw it away until the abcess has healed.

- If you develop cracked nipples, use a nipple shield every alternate feed and change the position of your baby so that the sucking is using different areas of your nipples each time. Take a mild analgesic, such as paracetamol, half-an-hour before a feed is due so that you are not tense in anticipation of the pain. Baby will not have to suck as hard to get the milk if you are relaxed.

- During the first few days until your milk comes in, your baby will receive colostrum. This yellow fluid is very rich and full of antibodies important for immunity. Allow no one to tell you that he requires supplementing with cows' milk at this stage. Cows' milk can cause allergies to develop in a very young baby. If your baby is not satisfied and cries all the time even when fed frequently, give him a bottle of plain boiled water – he may be thirsty!

- If you have to give up *don't* feel guilty. You have done your best for him.

Should your baby be too small or too ill to suck from you, it is possible to ensure your milk supply by using a breast pump and feeding him by bottle with the expressed milk. It is doubly important for poorly babies to receive breast milk, and often the staff on a special care baby unit will take spare milk from the 'milk bank' for these children.

The afterpains experienced by many new mothers are often as painful as labour contractions. When you are breastfeeding these may be particularly strong. However, they are a good sign that your uterus is contracting back to its original size, down behind your pubic bone. This is another good reason for breastfeeding.

A common mistake made by many new mothers is to pay every attention to their babies but totally neglect themselves. If you omit to perform your postnatal exercises at this stage you will regret it later. The midwife will give you a leaflet with a set of exercises, which should be performed daily. Tummy muscles are most likely to suffer during pregnancy and will no doubt be a bit flabby for a few months. The muscles of the pelvic floor following a vaginal delivery are stretched out of shape and require toning by exercise. This is especially important as you have successive children if you are to avoid prolapse of the womb at a later stage. When you go to the toilet to pass water, practise stopping the flow and then starting again, as a means of using the pelvic floor muscles. Once you know how this feels you can draw up these muscles without visiting the loo! Sleep on your stomach so that the uterus falls into its correct position and does not become retroverted (tilted backwards). Never strain your lower back muscles following a birth by trying to practise double leg raising; your stomach muscles are just not strong enough at this stage for that exercise. Regaining your correct posture is also of great importance. Backache from bending over can be a real nuisance to a new mother when lifting and carrying her infant. This can be avoided by following the advice on posture and remembering always to bend from the knees.

Any lacerations of the perineum or stitches should heal within a week of the birth. Salt baths with a handful of sage herbs added are a great aid to a healing perineum, and comfrey ointment can be used to reduce bruising. Many women are afraid to restart their sex life after giving birth. Until quite recently the advice given to women was that sex should not be attempted until six weeks after delivery. However, this is old-fashioned and unnecessary. Once the vagina is properly healed, and the lochia (vaginal loss following the birth) has diminished, gentle intercourse may be attempted. You should ensure that your vagina is well lubricated. This may require the use of lubricating jelly, especially as you may be tense the first couple of times.

Arriving home with a new baby is a pretty scary adventure for parents, especially if it is the first child. Expect nothing. Accept what happens, then deal with it. Expectations of a peacefully sleeping, clean infant who awakens at regular intervals to be fed and then goes straight back to sleep again are destined to be dashed. Babies are very contrary creatures with their own habits, moods and personality. If they cry constantly for even one day they drive you to distraction, as this plays on your fears of being a 'bad' parent who cannot cope with the child's demands. Forgive yourself 100 times a day for not being perfect!

Your relationship with your partner will inevitably come under some strain during this time. Many marriages founder on the rocks of parenthood, and this is very often because of lack of communication between the couple. The complete involvement from early pregnancy of both parents in planning for their offspring can alleviate many of the problems. Women inevitably tend to receive most of the attention during the pregnancy because of the biological factors. However the arrival of a baby creates a new family, and its survival as a unit will depend on sound co-operation between the adults of the household.

Start early by discussing your expectations of each other and yourselves as parents before you try to conceive your first child. Remember that your own upbringing and experience of being a child will have a bearing on the sort of behaviour you expect of yourself and your partner as parents. There are no holidays from children, and the commitment they require can be draining for even the most willing parent. A child is an individual born into the world where he or she has to learn to exist with other individuals. This learning process starts at birth and will be coloured by your behaviour as parents. Ensure that you are prepared to accept that responsibility as mature adult people before embarking on parenthood.

Common ailments of the new-born infant

Once you are left alone with your new child, without the regular attentions of your midwife, the full weight of responsibility falls on your shoulders as parents. This is exciting but may also feel quite a heavy burden, especially if you are feeling tired from constantly broken nights. If your baby becomes ill or cries frequently, you may feel downright panicky. However, there are many quite simple problems which are easy for you to deal with. Your health visitor should come to see you on at least a couple of occasions, hopefully to lend support and give advice on feeding problems.

We have given here a few examples of the more common of the problems experienced with new infants, with suggestions on how you might tackle them.

● *Jaundice.* This is a condition caused by immaturity of the liver and causes mild, yellow discolouration of the skin. Jaundiced babies often look as though they have a good suntan! Treatment, apart from extra fluids, is not necessary unless the condition is severe, in which case phototherapy is used. Mothers are asked to place their babies in the natural sunlight at a window whenever possible. As that is not often possible in this country, there are machines in the baby care units at hospitals to give the light artificially. Premature babies are most at risk from this condition, but full-term babies can be affected also.

● *Feeding problems.* These are often the result of faults in feeding technique by the parents, but can be due to illness. Very few are caused by the type of milk formula used, and frequent changes in the brand of milk are unnecessary.

Meddlesome interference by relatives or ill-informed nurses can account for many of the problems associated with breastfeeding. Some mothers are unaware that only colostrum is produced for the first two or three days before the breast milk 'comes in'.

The commonest fault with bottlefeeding is mechanical, caused when too large or too small a hole is used in the teat. This causes the baby to swallow large amounts of air with the milk, which produces a distended stomach and subsequent vomiting. Overfeeding very frequently creates problems for the bottlefed new baby. This is sometimes deliberate, as an attempt to stop crying, or by incorrect mixing of the milk formula.

● *Vomiting.* This is usually a symptom of overfeeding, but it can also be due to an infection. Simple 'mouthing' of small quantities of milk is quite normal in a very young baby. Infections, such as a cold, are the commonest cause of persistent vomiting.

Vomiting may also be due to immaturity of the valve situated at the junction between the stomach and the gullet, which fails to stay closed when the stomach becomes full. The milk is then regurgitated and is known as 'reflux'. This is cured very simply by thickening the feed with special granules. A feed should never be thickened by adding extra scoops of milk powder formula.

A more rare condition, known as pyloric stenosis, may cause persistent projectile vomiting. This is caused by an obstruction at the outlet of the stomach and is cured by surgery.

● *Diarrhoea*. The essential characteristic of the diarrhoeal stool is that it is very runny with an excess of watery fluid. The colour and frequency are not usually important. Feeding problems and milk formula are rarely causative factors. Diarrhoea is more commonly caused by infection, either caught from another infected person or by poor hygiene.

Profuse diarrhoea in a small baby is potentially dangerous, as there is the possibility of dehydration developing. This is diagnosed by the child's poor skin texture, dry mouth, feeble cry and apathy. Hospital admission is frequently necessary. However, if diarrhoea is mild, it is usually sufficient to stop all milk and solid feeds and just give the baby liberal amounts of fluid. A mixture of one teaspoon of salt, five teaspoons of sugar and one pint of boiled water is recommended to stave off dehydration. In a young baby of less than three months, the strength of this solution should be reduced by half. It is possible to buy this mixture in powder formula to be added to water.

● *Constipation*. During the first few weeks, a breastfed baby will produce stools the colour and consistency of mustard in almost every nappy. The frequency of these will reduce as the baby matures, and the baby may go for several days without a bowel movement with no ill effects. A bottlefed baby will have darker, smellier, harder stools once or twice a day.

Genuine constipation doesn't usually happen until solid food is introduced into the diet. This is usually signalled by difficulty in evacuating very hard stools and is often accompanied by slight bleeding. Treatment is usually dietary and should include extra fresh fruit, vegetables, plus fruit juices and extra water to which a little sugar may be added. Purgatives should be rigorously avoided.

● *Colic*. The irritable baby is often labelled 'colicky'. It is possibly significant that 'colic' almost always happens around six o'clock in the evening when the mother is trying to prepare an evening meal, bath the baby and see to other tired children before bedtime!

It is not unreasonable to assume that it may be due to aerophagis (swallowing of air) because of over-eager feeding or poor technique. A very hungry baby is more likely to gulp his feed and suffer colic if he has been left to cry for a long time before the feed.

Immunisation

This subject is a minefield of emotional and ethical problems. Over the past few years the debate has raged about the advantages and disadvantages of immunisation. There is no arguing with the facts which state that the deadly disease smallpox has been eradicated from the face of the earth by worldwide vaccination programmes. The large isolation hospitals and sanitoriums for infectious diseases no longer exist. Although there are some very unfortunate cases of children becoming brain-damaged following vaccination, the children whose lives have been blighted by severe infectious diseases are rarely mentioned in the counter-argument. This is quite apart from the horrible suffering encountered during the illness, and those who actually die of complications.

Contra-indications to immunisations (i.e. when not to immunise) are:

- Any child who is currently suffering from an acute infectious disease.
- Prematurity (vaccination should be appropriately delayed).
- Children with defective immune systems (a rare condition).
- Any child who had a severe reaction to the first dose of vaccine.
- A child with an allergy to eggs should not be immunised against measles as the vaccine is cultured on eggs.
- Any child who has a neurological impairment or an abnormality such as 'jitteriness' following a difficult birth or brain damage at birth; who has epilepsy or has a close relative suffering from epilepsy (parent or sibling); or who has had a major reaction to a previous vaccine should *not* be immunised against whooping cough.

No one can advise you as a parent what to do about having your child vaccinated. Once you know both sides of the argument you can make your own decisions. Don't allow other people to make your decisions for you, as you are the parents responsible for that child and it is you who have to look after them for the foreseeable future. Ensure that you are well informed as to the nature of the disease, its possible consequence, and the current figures for vaccine-related brain damage.

Immunisation Table

4–6 months	1st triple antigen (diphtheria, whooping cough, tetanus)
	1st polio
6–8 months	2nd triple
	2nd polio
1 year	3rd triple
	MMR (measles, mumps, rubella)
	3rd polio
4½–5 years	booster diphtheria, tetanus
	booster polio

Tetanus and polio vaccinations should be repeated every five years.

Milestones
As we have stressed throughout this book, every person is an individual in their own right and will develop entirely at their own rate. Competition is rife between parents as to how intelligent, talented and advanced their own offspring are – from the first smile onwards! This competition can easily be felt as pressure to 'perform' by even very young children.

Unfortunately, some of the staff at developmental clinics reinforce this attitude by 'failing' children on their tests if they do not perform a certain task correctly on a set day. In fact, it is a trend over a period of time which matters rather than one result on a particular day. Continual comparison of children can lead to labelling them as 'failures' or 'winners' for life, and may not allow them room to display their own talents or shortcomings if they are boxed into a specific category.

It is with this in mind that you must approach the developmental sessions at the clinic. Remember that if your child was born prematurely or was poorly after birth, this will have had some effect on his rate of development. The following table is to help your awareness of what the assessor is looking for in your child.

Development Table

Height and weight are measured at each session.

1 week	Feeding ability. Exclusion of congenital abnormalities. Blood test screening for phenylketonuria.
6 weeks	Response to mother. Smiling and gaze fixation. Stilling of cry in response to mother's voice. Presence of simple reflexes such as grasp reflex. (These early reflexes disappear within a few weeks.)
6 months	Social responses such as babbling and smiling. Hand and eye co-ordination, early manipulation ability (i.e. being able to pick up and hold small objects). Motor control: sitting, good head control, ability to take weight on legs. Hearing tests.
18 months–2 years	Social skills: recognition of parts of the body. Response to questions and simple instructions. Involvement in play. Walking ability. Hearing tests. Control of bowels at two years. Sight tests.
3-3½ years	Explorative play, free conversation and simple sentences. Listening to stories. Imitating behaviour. Progressive control of bladder and bowels. Sight tests.

4-4½ years Running and climbing. Active, social and imaginative play. Ability to draw and colour. Normal speech. Full bladder and bowel control. Sight tests.

If you are fortunate, the doctors and health visitors who perform these tests will be sensitive to your needs and concerns as parents and will not alarm you unnecessarily about any adverse results. The whole point of these exercises is to ensure that your child does not have any disability which could be prevented from developing and causing him to be disadvantaged among his contemporaries.

Weaning

Along with potty training, this is one of the main bones of contention among parents! Unfortunately, fashions come and go every few years and not many of these take into account the individual nature of the children concerned. You will be offered plenty of advice, and probably not much of it will be relevant to your baby. Professional advice is often inflexible and unhelpful. We have seen mothers almost at breaking-point because they have an unhappy, hungry baby who is obviously in need of extra solid food but whose health visitor is sticking to rigid rules of advice. A very small amount of solid food can also settle the 'windy' baby who is only six weeks old or so. The following set of loose guidelines might help you decide whether your baby is ready to be weaned.

- If your baby was over nine pounds at birth and is not satisfied between feeds once he reaches 12 to 14 pounds.
- Once he reaches the stage where he needs feeding every two-and-a-half to three hours with milk.
- If he starts to wake more frequently during the night for extra food.
- Once he reaches three to four months, if none of the other points apply before this stage.

It is up to you which meal give your baby first, according to the routine you have. The important rule is never to feed a baby immediately before a bath, and remember that small babies often feel too tired after a bath to do full justice to a solid meal. We are in great favour of introducing babies to a feeder cup (a cup with a lid which has a small spout with holes through which to drink), as this helps them to learn to drink by themselves rather than being fed, so encouraging independence and saving unnecessary spillage!

By six months you will probably be aiming to have your child on three meals a day so that he will fit in with your own routine. The following is an example of how you might like to plan the day at that stage so that when you start weaning you know what you are aiming at!

Suggested feeding plan for six-month-old baby

7 am	Breast or bottle feed.
8.30 am	Cereal and fruit breakfast. Juice drink.
12 midday	Lunch. Thick vegetable broth. Yoghurt. Breast or bottle feed.
4 pm	Tea. Mashed ripe avocado or puréed fruit. Juice.
6.30 pm	Breast or bottle feed.

These times and suggested foods are only a rough guide. Your own plan will depend very much on what time your baby wakes and whether you have to go out to work or have other children to attend to. As you progress you will probably drop the lunchtime feed and substitute a cup of boiled milk or juice. (Do not use milk in a feeder cup as it is not possible to clean the holes in the spout properly, so creating a medium in which bacteria can easily grow.) Retaining the feeds in the early morning and evening are useful for comfort purposes.

If your baby is on three meals a day plus two other feeds, he will not require night feeds. This does not mean that he will not ask for them! If you have had enough of broken nights, try substituting very weak juice and then boiled water for evening milk feed. This often helps to get the message across! It is quite fair to feel you have some right to some unbroken sleep and amazing how much better you are able to cope once you have a few nights of sleep. A note of warning: Babies often cry for comfort, although it feels like the little dears are being awkward in the extreme! Ignoring this plea for love and comfort can have an adverse effect in the long term. A baby who has been cuddled and attended to has a better chance of growing into an emotionally secure and independent toddler.

Your baby will enjoy some foods and not others, so you have to use trial and error as to which ones to use. Baby rice is the usual starter food recommended for weaning babies as it can be mixed with milk. Start the good habits early. Ensure that there is no added sugar or salt, and that there are no chemical flavourings, preservatives or colourings in the food. Make a habit of reading the labels on all the food you buy for the family. Chemical additives are often responsible for hyperactivity and allergies such as asthma and eczema in young children. Some children have definite allergies or dislikes to certain foods, so if you are introducing a new food be alert for any adverse reactions such as a rash, irritability or wakefulness.

Weaning a baby is the perfect opportunity to start the whole family on a healthier diet. This should ideally be of the low-fat, high-fibre variety. Puréed fruit and vegetables make marvellous meals for your baby. Always use the freshest produce and never use any food which has signs of mould. In particular, do not use potatoes which have green patches in them. Keep the stock after you have boiled vegetables (not potatoes) and use it to make soups with the addition of more vegetables and pulses such as lentils. These can be liquidised to a smooth consistency for a small baby. Remember that most cheeses contain salt and are quite high in fat content, so cottage cheese is a much better option. Natural yoghurts are a wonderful ready meal and a good source of calcium, which can be found in both sheep's and goats' milk varieties as well as cows'. Mashed fruit, such as bananas, can be added to this to vary the taste. Ripe avocados and papaya fruits are also ready-made meals.

Once your baby has some teeth or gums hard enough to eat 'finger foods', rusks and slices of fruit make easy and nutritious teas. Rusks can be made with thick, finger slices of wholemeal bread baked at a low temperature in the oven. Always stay with your child throughout the meal when he is feeding himself, as it only takes a few seconds for him to choke. Save feeding your baby eggs until he is nine months old or so, as these are thought to be responsible for encouraging allergies in an immature gut. Although tinned, and packaged foods are second-rate compared to freshly prepared meals, they are very useful if you are busy. Try to keep them in reserve for occasions when you have absolutely no time to make a fresh meal.

Introduce meat in stages by first giving carefully boned fish, then chicken and, lastly, small amounts of red meat once or twice a week. Do not worry about having to flavour the food, as what seems bland to you will be very tasty to children due to the fact that they have more taste buds than adults. Stick to fresh fruit juices with a little added boiled water for drinks rather than paying for bottled squash drinks which are often loaded with sugar and chemical additives. Boiled cows' milk can be given from the age of six months onwards, but as this can be responsible for over production of mucus it shouldn't be given at every meal.

CHILDHOOD

Staying with the good habits

If you have read the earlier chapter on food and diet, you will have the information on how to start eating a healthier diet and how to stick with it. Be wary of being a hypocrite by trying to feed your kids a healthy diet while you eat the chips and chocolate! Children are not easily fooled and will copy your habits. The main aim is to educate your children in healthy eating habits so that when they are old enough to choose their own food they will pick what is good for them and enjoy it. When they are very young, as parents you will have almost total control over what they consume. However, as they grow and become more independent you will have less and less say over what they eat, especially when they start school. (This is where your teaching and encouragement will pay off.) If your child has fresh fruit after every meal, then he will no doubt continue this habit with his school meals.

Your child will, inevitably, try out new tastes and flavours which have hitherto been absent at home. For instance, we never had a bottle of tomato ketchup in our house until our eldest child started school dinners. He took a liking to this new flavour and, rather than begin a battle with him, we agreed to buy some. However, there are so few meals in our household which go with ketchup that it rarely makes an appearance on the table!

We have found that with some children, if a certain item (whether it be food, a television programme or a toy) is absolutely banned they become almost obsessed by it, and so begins an ugly battle of wills. Our own plan has been to allow whatever it is they want (within reason of safety and finances), but explain why we are not keen on their idea. Take chocolate as an example. Visitors often bring chocolate or sweets to the house for the children. We allow them some of it and keep the rest for other days. It is also kept out of reach of small fingers, where there is no temptation to keep going back to it. Similarly with fizzy drinks, these have to be asked for rather than the children being able to help themselves. Conversely, fruit juices, bread, fresh fruit and other healthy nibbles are kept at their level in the cupboards so that they can help themselves. Rather than totally denying the 'junk' food such as beefburgers and chips, allow children these every now and again, being careful not to make them appear special in any way.

Crisps have been a controversial food item, provoking different opinions as to whether they are good for you or not. They are, in fact, high in fibre and vitamin C. However, in the main potato crisps have a high fat content, usually with added salt and flavouring. The manufacturers have realised this and you can now buy low-fat, unflavoured crisps. Some health shops also sell a variety of 'natural' rather than chemically flavoured crisps.

Try not to forget to stress the positive effects of your child's healthier diet to him occasionally. These are that he is ill less often and also able to shrug off any sickness quicker than those of his friends who are not eating healthily, which will no doubt be the case!

There are several wholefood cookery books available which contain suggestions for children's food. The following are some tips we have picked up in our attempts to feed our three children a healthy diet.

- Make the food look interesting by arranging it in shapes such as faces, spaceships and monsters.
- Most children seem to adore pasta. This makes a wonderful easy and nutritious meal when the wholewheat variety is used.
- Become expert at 'hiding' foods which your child dislikes, e.g. liquidise essential greens in a purée, soup or filling of a pie.
- Always look out for the healthier alternative, e.g. baked beans without sugar, or oven chips with less fat.
- Avoid straight confrontation about food whenever possible. Food has a very high emotional value and can be used as a weapon quite easily by the youngest of children, as well as parents.
- As we suggested in the chapter on food and diet, become a regular label reader so that you are aware of what is hidden in food, and be especially wary of products which are labelled 'natural' as this doesn't mean anything in health terms.

We believe that this positive approach encourages children to enjoy their food and helps them to distinguish what is 'good' and what is 'bad' without making an issue out of every meal or creating problem habits. This should also engender a balanced sense of choice for the child as they are not being denied 'forbidden fruit'.

Common childhood ailments

Once your child starts to attend a toddler group, playgroup or school he will undoubtedly catch some of the infectious diseases associated with childhood. The more serious ones, such as whooping cough and measles, can be vaccinated against (see page 88). However, colds, stomach upsets and other viral infections will probably be encountered from time to time. Hopefully your child will be fit enough to resist the majority of these and will gain immunity as time goes by. A healthy child should throw off the worst effects of most of these diseases within a few days.

It is always a worry if your child seems off-colour or becomes ill. As a general rule, always take your child to a doctor if he becomes drowsy or lethargic. A high temperature signifies the body's defence to an infection. High fevers can cause convulsions in some small children, which are alarming to say the least. However, these are not a sign of epilepsy and are termed 'febrile' convulsions. If your child has a very high temperature, cool him gradually by tepid sponging and ensure that he is not wrapped in blankets or too many layers of clothing. Paracetamol syrup will also help to reduce the fever.

● *Coughing.* This is commonly caused by viral infection of the upper respiratory tract, and is a protective reflex which prevents mucus blocking the airway.

Hot drinks of lemon and honey are soothing and do much to relieve the discomfort of coughing. Camphorated oil can be rubbed into the chest at night in order to aid breathing. Steam inhalations of friars balsam help to break up the mucus.

● *Asthma.* Persistent night coughing with wheezing should alert you to the possibility of asthma and a medical opinion should be sought. The incidence of asthma has increased over the past 10 years and up to 6 per cent of all children are affected to some degree.

The condition manifests because of tightening of the

airways due to a combination of allergy, infection and certain emotional states such as excitement or upset. This leads to wheezing and progressive problems with inhaling enough air for the body's functions. It can be relieved with the use of a simple inhaler or nebuliser (a special machine which may be used safely at home and usually prevents hospital admission). Preventative measures are much preferred, and may include allergy testing in order to avoid contact with allergenic substances, physiotherapy to improve breathing technique, and avoidance of high emotional states.

Any persistent cough in a child should be checked, especially in young babies, to rule out the possibility of chest infection such as bronchitis.

● *Whooping cough.* Controversy over the rare complications associated with vaccination against this miserable disease has overshadowed the true mortality rate before vaccination was available. Infants up to the age of one year are most at risk from suffering serious complications from whooping cough, the major one of which is pneumonia. This illness appears in cycles, becoming epidemic once every four years.

The child will appear catarrhal for three days, subsequently developing coughing spasms which can last up to 30 minutes. These are characterised by a series of whoops as the child desperately tries to breathe. There may also be some blood coughed up in the sputum. Treatment is limited and mainly supportive.

● *Throat and ear infections.* Ninety per cent of these are viral in origin and therefore do not require an antibiotic. Earache is usually due to blockage of the eustachian tube (the passageway between the ear and the back of the throat) by mucus. If the ear is discharging, then an antibiotic is usually needed. Painkillers (without aspirin) can be given to relieve the pain.

Sore throats can be relieved by copious amounts of warm fruit drinks and painkillers if necessary. If the child is old enough, he might gargle with a weak solution of salt.

● *Diarrhoea and vomiting*. The cause of this problem is most commonly infection. Antibiotics should never be given as they reduce the body's own defences and worsen the symptoms. Always seek a medical opinion when a child under three has severe diarrhoea and vomiting, because of the threat of dehydration.

The older child should be starved for 24 hours and only given sips of plain spring water or boiled tap water. After this period a couple of spoonfuls of 'live' plain yoghurt can be given to boost the immune system in the gut. Diluted fresh fruit juices may be administered as necessary. As the child recovers, you might give him some plain boiled rice or a banana. Only give small amounts until you are sure the vomiting has ceased.

● *Urine infections*. These are usually found in girls, due to the fact that they have a straight, short urethra (small front passage leading from the bladder) so germs easily find their way into the urinary tract. The child will complain on passing water and may pass some blood in the urine. In babies there may be no specific symptoms apart from a pale appearance and poor feeding.

Cystitis usually requires treatment with antibiotics, and copious fluids to dilute the acidity of the urine. If the symptoms are recurrent then investigations may be necessary in order to rule out kidney problems.

● *Measles*. Measles is a very nasty viral disease which can make the child feel quite poorly. Complications, although rare, can be very serious and include conjunctivitis, photophobia, pneumonia, loss of hearing, reduced eyesight, meningitis and, in very serious cases, death. The incubation period is 8 to 14 days after infection.

The illness begins with symptoms similar to a cold: general malaise, sore throat and watery eyes. A generalised, florid rash, commencing at the hairline, appears within three days of the initial symptoms.

● *Rubella (German measles)*. This is usually a mild disease with little effect on the general health. The child may complain of cold symptoms for a day or so but there will be no conjunctivitis or other complications present. Classically, the patient will have enlarged glands at the back of the neck and a pale rash for three or four days. This disease can sometimes be so mild that the child and parents are unaware that rubella is present. If you are aware that other children in the district have this illness, be particularly wary of mixing with them if you are pregnant or have contact with other pregnant women who have no immunity to rubella. (See section on pre-pregnancy.)

● *Mumps*. You will probably be in little doubt if your child contracts mumps, as he will look something like a hamster with full cheeks! The incubation period is anything from two weeks to a full month after infection. The child may complain of pain when eating for a day or so and the side of the face will be tender to touch on one or both sides. This should not be confused with simple swelling of the neck glands. A mild fever is usually present. In theory, the younger the child the less serious mumps is, as complications involving the testicles can occur after puberty. This has been known to lead to sterility in severe cases.

● *Chicken pox*. This is a particularly infectious but usually mild disease. As with the other viral infections, your child will probably be ill with a temperature for a day or so, though it is possible that you will not realise he has chicken pox until the first spot appears. The incubation period is 12 to 16 days. On the first day only a few single spots erupt, but this rapidly increases on the second and third days until the trunk is covered. These lesions can be extremely unpleasant and very itchy. They progress from a raised, red lump to a pustule, finally drying into a scab. Calamine lotion often eases the itching to some extent. Chicken pox is infectious for a couple of days before and one week after the day the first spot appears.

- *Hyperactivity*. Classically, this child has a very short attention span, is constantly restless and sleeps for very short spells. He often has aggressive and destructive tendencies which culminate in serious learning and social problems.

Food allergies and high IQs are known to be causative factors in hyperactivity, but the commonest cause is the disturbed family unit. Medicine has very little part to play and therapy with a psychologist is usually required. If your child has periods of hyperactivity, take care to notice what he has eaten or drunk in the previous few hours. Chocolate, tartrazine (a colorant used in orange drinks) and fizzy drinks containing caffeine are often responsible for 'manic' behaviour in children.

These are some of the more common childhood illnesses which you are likely to come into contact with once you are a parent. If you are ever in doubt about the health of your child, always seek a medical opinion in order to put your mind at rest, even if this is only a telephone consultation.

GROWING UP – AND AWAY

Two of life's more painful lessons are learning that your parents are not perfect, and learning that you as a parent are not perfect either. Each generation swears they will not make the same mistakes as their parents, and they rarely do. There are a whole lot of other mistakes to be made and learned from!

Once your child reaches puberty, there are many new problems to be faced which can create difficulties for the whole family. No matter how well prepared you feel you are to cope with an adolescent, there will always be an experience waiting to surprise you. This will probably be linked to your own feelings and values, which are going to be severely tested and questioned during this phase.

Some of our most closely guarded and personal emotions are those concerning sex and our own sexuality. The adolescent phase is the time when sexuality develops and becomes apparent physically, mentally and emotionally. Most parents are approaching middle age as their offspring reach puberty. This situation often leads to jealousy, as the time when the next generation is setting out on life's great adventure is when your generation is coming to terms with mortality and ageing. It can be a trying and confusing time for teenagers and parents alike.

A healthy, stable teenager will test his boundaries to the limits while still needing to be shown that he is loved and cared about. Letting go of a beloved child and encouraging independence is a gradual process which begins at birth and reaches its critical stage during adolescence. There are likely to be rather fewer confrontations in the family where the child has been allowed room to develop as an individual, play a part in decision-making and encouraged to take responsibility for his actions, than in one where parents have been autocratic. The bridge between child- and adulthood can be rickety and even dangerous, but it is a process which may also be adventurous: full of rewarding experiences and bitter-sweet memories to savour.

There are particular types of stress experienced by teenagers which are of little relevance to other age groups. Depending upon the individual character of the teenager, he will usually come under pressure from a dilemma concerning one of the following areas.

Educational pressures

Puberty, especially in girls, can often begin as young as 10 years old, even before they leave junior school. The pressures of beginning at a new, larger senior school can be quite unnerving for the average 11-year-old. Exams and their results are a feature of adolescence which many of us would rather forget. The brightest of children can fail in exams under the pressure to 'do well' from both parents and teachers who require good results in order to make themselves look good.

Conflicts often arise over the choice between social occasions and schoolwork. Children taking GCSEs and A level courses are often loaded down with homework necessary to cover the syllabus, at a time when learning social skills is of great importance to their emotional development.

Sexual pressures

If you have answered all your child's questions about sex honestly and openly as they have arisen from an early age, then he will no doubt be less confused than a child whose embarrassed parents have avoided giving straightforward answers. Your child will feel able to continue approaching you with questions pertaining to sexual matters if you have laid the foundations by accepting his questions and dealing with them matter-of-factly.

Whereas the early questions were probably rather mechanical and technical, those posed after the age of 11 or so will be much more complex, involving the emotional and moral viewpoints. As your child grows up it is going to become more difficult for you, as a parent, actually to have control over his behaviour. With this in mind, give your child the facts and then discuss the pros and cons of certain types of sexual and social behaviour. Hopefully, this route will help your teenager to come to his own considered decisions. He will not always reach the decision you would have liked! There are bound to be some heated moments.

● *Periods.*
Some girls start their periods as early as 10, and many by the age of 11 years. Prepare your daughter for menstruation by explaining what actually happens and the reasons why she will bleed each month. We all know what a nuisance periods can be, so it is worth stressing the positive points to someone who is about to embark on years of menstruation. Enable her to realise that she is approaching womanhood and preparing to be able to carry a baby inside her eventually.

● *Crushes.*
Infatuation with a distant person is often experienced during puberty. The object of desire can often be a pop star, television personality or teacher, and is frequently a person of the same sex. This kind of infatuation is a safe way of dealing with what can be violent passion. Many teenagers will develop close, sometimes sexual relationships with a member of their own sex and, although a certain percentage of adolescents will remain homosexual or bisexual, the majority pass through this stage in their early teens.

● *Masturbation.*
Many children masturbate from an early age and continue into adulthood. However, as sexual feelings surface during puberty it becomes more likely that the adolescent will experiment with masturbation to relieve sexual needs. There is certainly no danger to health in this perfectly natural habit, and it is obviously much safer for a young teenager than experimentation with sexual partners. It is now known that cervical cancer is more likely to occur in a woman who started having sexual intercourse before the age of 16.

● *Safe sex.*
The dilemma for many parents is how to warn children of the dangers associated with certain types of sexual practice without frightening them off making relationships and enjoying a subsequent happy sexual relationship. It may also be difficult to discuss the many emotional and physical problems linked with sex without appearing to condone promiscuous sexual behaviour. Often children will rebel directly against parents' instructions as they feel they are old enough not to be 'told' what to do. Let your kids know all the facts – good and bad. Give them your own opinions about the facts along with the reasons why you hold those views, and be prepared to have your ideas challenged. Above all, *be there* if they need to talk to you and listen to what they are saying to you. Accepting one's children's developing sexuality is

probably almost as difficult as coming to terms with the fact that your parents are also sexual beings! Denying them their sexuality and growing maturity may cause them to go out and have it accepted elsewhere.

We consider that it is worth telling your children about contraception before they are likely to experience a sexual relationship, at, say, the age of 12 or 13. This could be linked into a general conversation about their changing bodies and why these changes are happening. A description of what occurs during puberty easily leads into the mechanical descriptions of how pregnancy occurs and how it might be prevented. Remember to put the same emphasis on preventing pregnancies to your sons as well as to your daughters.

It is unfortunate that the 'swinging sixties' have left a swingeing legacy for the next generation. Herpes, AIDS and the high incidence of cervical cancer have created a new set of problems for the young. One wonders whether they will rebel against their parents' generation by remaining celibate!

Safe sex is only possible with a monogamous partner who has no recent history of other intimate relationships. Safer sex involves avoiding oral sex and any other practice which involves exchange of body fluids (urine, semen and vaginal secretions). The use of a condom is an absolute must during intercourse with a partner whose history you are not sure of, in order to decrease the chances of spreading sexually transmitted diseases.

Most adolescents will attempt 'petting' before they have full intercourse with a partner. This will carry some risk of disease-spreading. For instance, if the petting should involve the boy putting his fingers into the girl's vagina, when he has a cut on his finger she could receive the AIDS virus from his blood or he could receive it from her if the vaginal fluid enters the cut.

Sexual feelings are very potent during adolescence and teenagers are rather at the mercy of their hormone levels. Once your nearly adult teenager is sexually active, he will be less willing to heed your warnings. He may well see you as a spoilsport, bent on moralising and curbing his enjoyment. For this reason we suggest that you try to talk about the dangers of disease when your child is around the age of 13 and 14, depending of course, upon how mature he is for his age.

Although this is not widely known, cervical cancer is now considered to be directly related to the number of partners a woman has had and how early she started having intercourse. The earlier intercourse begins and the higher the number of partners, the larger the risk of developing cancer of the cervix. Genital warts are known to be a major cause of this type of cancer and can be caught during unprotected intercourse with an infected man. Once your daughter has become sexually active, she should have a cervical smear every two to three years up to the age of 35, after which time this should be performed every year.

Help your daughter to develop the good habit of examining her own breasts for lumps each month after her period has finished. This should be done by raising one arm above her head and, using the flat of the hand, pressing into the breast tissue under the arm and working around the breast until all of it has been covered. This exercise should then be repeated on the other side.

Misuse of drugs

As these teenage years are a time of exploration of the wider world, there are unfortunate situations along with the positive experiences to be encountered. Cigarettes, alcohol and other drugs are available for experimentation. Your child may well come under pressure to try one or more of these substances. Children as young as seven are known to have been coaxed into trying hard drugs such as cocaine or heroin. It is extremely unlikely that this will happen to your child, but it is worth being aware of the dangers of drug pedlars at the school gates.

Simple hazards such as leaving the drinks cupboard unlocked or a packet of cigarettes lying around may encourage a child to 'have a go'. This may sound as though it could lead to a comic situation, but in fact it is extremely dangerous.

Alcohol is a poison, and children have died from accidental overdosing. Likewise, the dangers of fire are apparent if a young child tries lighting a cigarette.

Glue sniffing has been highlighted as the drug of young teenagers because of its availability and cheapness. Fortunately, legislation has meant that solvents cannot be sold to children under 18, but children can be devious and may ask an older person to buy it for them on pretext.

The tell-tale signs of drug abuse in teenagers are difficult to spot, mainly because they are not very far removed from normal adolescent behaviour. However, if you know your child well you should be able to spot a change in the usual behaviour pattern. Be alert to lying or stealing, a neglected appearance, the need for junk food (hence the term 'junkie') and extreme apathy. Violent mood swings often indicate drug involvement. The child may well begin to smoke cigarettes. If you suspect your child is taking drugs, talk to his teachers, your GP and possibly his friends or their parents to find out if they have noticed any difference in behaviour.

It is possible that he may have experimented a couple of times with certain illegal substances but is not dependent upon them. Addiction is a slow, downhill process which progresses over a period of time. If it is caught early, it is possible to find help and a total cure reasonably simple, provided the child is amenable. Long-term drug abuse is much more difficult to cope with. Be aware that the willpower to cease use of a particular drug has to come from the addicted person. Your role is one of support. Again, education is necessary *before* the hazard presents itself, from, say, seven or eight years old. This may well help to prevent the problem from occurring at all, and is preferable to seeking a cure when some damage may already have been done. Counselling will involve a process of talking out the child's problems and trying to identify the emotional need for using drugs.

This problem is an increasing and malignant one within our society. Drug abuse is not confined to a particular group of people or social class. The havoc it wreaks upon families is appalling, ridden with guilt, anger and rejection for all the parties concerned. Although there are no absolute rules for avoiding drug dependence, a child who is raised to respect himself and his body is less likely to want to play with this type of fire than a child who is insecure and lacks self-respect.

Anorexia and bulimia

This distressing condition is confined mainly to the female gender and more specifically to teenage girls. An anorexic will simply starve herself, telling her parents at mealtimes that she has eaten already. Bulimia is similar, though characterised by periods of fasting punctuated by eating binges where the girl will eat enormous amounts of food and subsequently make herself vomit, only to start eating again. It is very much bound up with emotional issues and the girl's feelings about herself.

Anorexia nervosa may occur when a girl is developing her secondary sexual characteristics and begins menstruating. By starving herself she can stay boyishly thin and her periods will cease. This has obvious links to her fears of becoming adult and accepting sexual maturity. Once again, awareness of your daughter's development and acceptance of her approaching maturity may well help her to cope with these fears. Social pressures to remain stick-thin in order to be fashionable are quite high, and often have a strong effect upon a fashion-conscious teenager.

In recent years, research has shown that people who are deficient in zinc are prone to develop anorexia. As zinc is most readily available in red meat, vegetarians are most at risk. A simple test whereby a specific chemical solution is dropped on to the tongue will prove whether the patient is zinc-deficient or not. To someone whose levels of zinc are normal the solution tastes appalling, whereas it has no taste for a person whose zinc levels are low. Although zinc levels have obvious positive connotations for the sufferers of anorexia, counselling or psychotherapy are usually an integral part of treatment.

Acne

Severe acne can often make a teenager miserable and withdrawn. It is a very common problem, particularly in boys, and is linked to changing hormone levels which increase the skin's acidity, causing irritation.

Treatment includes attention to diet with a high intake of fresh raw fruit and vegetables, plus copious amounts of mineral water each day. Natural sunlight, as opposed to artificial ultraviolet light, is helpful, and acne frequently improves during the summer months. Sulphur tablets are useful for cleansing the system and often help to improve the condition. Unfortunately, acne does become worse when the sufferer is under stress. In extreme cases a low-dose antibiotic is prescribed for long periods, and is often preferable to scarring both the skin and the tender teenage ego.

MARRIAGE AND LIVING TOGETHER

Although this is not an inevitable lifestage, most people do eventually select and settle down with a (supposedly) permanent life partner. Due to their extremely complex nature, it is unrealistic to expect to examine all the emotional issues concerned with adult male–female relationships in this short section of the book. However, we feel it is worth commenting on some of the more crucial matters concerned because of the close association between emotional and physical health.

Marriage can be heaven or hell and most long-term marriage partners would admit to having experienced both extremes during their time together. Our expectations of a chosen life partner are generally very high, because of the hope of having our emotional, sexual and material needs met by one human being. In fact, we look outwards for gratification which has to be found within ourselves. In its best form, marriage is an ideal arena in which the old, learned feelings and responses may be replayed and explored in order to find growth and healing and to gain love of oneself and one's partner through mutual trust, respect and understanding. A person who learns to love him- or herself is a lovable and loving being.

A one-in-three divorce rate may seem alarming, but in fact marriage has never been more popular. Many of those who have divorced marry a second or even third time in their search for happiness. Those couples who go into marriage young are most likely to become the casualties of the divorce statistics. This, in the main, is because the rate of growth and change in attitudes and outlook is more rapid in youth, and gradually slows with maturity. Conversely, a mature couple who have lived single lives for many years, only pleasing themselves, may be too entrenched in their ways to allow them to make the compromises necessary in a close relationship.

Throughout this book we have mentioned how expectation and reality often differ greatly. Many a starry-eyed young couple have rushed headlong into a permanent relationship only to be rudely awakened by the realities of living together after the honeymoon is over. The ceremony and traditions surrounding the marriage service frequently overshadow the importance of the relationship between bride and groom. The search for a home, its subsequent furnishing and all the preparations for the wedding day are the main focus of attention, and often detract from the emotional state of play between the couple in question. Some people are more in love with the idea they have of marriage than they are with their real prospective partner, although they don't realise it. In the case of young couples, conflict with parents often drives them to seek a marriage partner and leads straight into another unhappy situation.

Many people find it very difficult to define why they love someone. For this reason it is not always easy to rationalise how or why these feelings change when they 'fall out of love'. Apart from the obvious practical factors such as avoiding loneliness, monetary considerations and rearing a family, there are underlying emotional needs as to why one person is attracted to another. These hidden elements become important when a relationship starts to falter. A crisis within a marriage is often triggered by a major life event such as those which have been detailed in this chapter. The birth of a child, death of a parent, loss of a job or moving to a new home, indeed any happening which changes the usual pattern of life, is likely to stir feelings in one or both partners about themselves and their roles within the marriage. A common example is that in which one partner has played 'parent' to the other. The birth of a child into that family is likely to cause a shift in the status quo creating possible jealousy or anger in the ousted 'child'.

When a major upheaval occurs, creating or revealing a marital crisis, there exists a marvellous opportunity to learn about yourself and your partner and so achieve emotional growth. The process requires self-honesty, with the need to delve into your own responses in relation to your partner. All of us have parts of our personality which are stunted because of what occurred during our development. When we experience a traumatic spell, our safety valve is often the ability to talk out our problems. This would seem to be a defensive mechanism designed to keep us healthy, as unexpressed negative feelings are often the cause of depression or physical illness in the long term. Research into the personality types of cancer victims has shown that they are often people who find it difficult to express their feelings and tend to bury them.

Emotional exploration is often a painful business, and involves accepting parts of yourself which are unpleasant and which you would rather deny existed. However, a thorough knowledge of yourself, of both your good and bad parts, will enable you to function better as a whole person, giving you some insight into why certain things happen in your life. This enables you to have a choice in your attitudes and behaviour, rather than feeling that events 'just happen' in your life. Our minds and bodies are basically programmed towards health. Patterns emerge constantly in our lives from which we can learn and grow towards wholeness, if we allow it to happen.

Though it is often the only way forward in many cases, divorce is an extremely painful process which entails feelings of guilt, anger and recrimination for all the parties concerned. It is also likely to have a profound effect upon the lives of any children involved. If this should happen to your marriage, take the opportunity to learn about *why* it happened to you, so that you can live more peacefully with yourself and with what is certain to be, at the least, a painful memory.

Contraception

The prevention or creation of a new human being is one of the most hotly debated aspects of human sexuality. In many religious and political systems the creation of children is zealously encouraged. In societies where this is so, contraception can be at best haphazard and at worst illegal. This is perhaps unfortunate in a world of finite, ever-diminishing resources and it must be the responsibility of every (hetero)-sexually active human being to consider their actions whenever they make love.

There is no perfect contraceptive in existence. The choice as to which suits your needs best and seems to have fewest disadvantages to your health and your enjoyment is a very individual one.

● *Contraceptive pill.*
Although there is no doubt about its convenience and effectiveness as a contraceptive measure, there is just as little doubt that the pill produces side-effects in a minority of users. These can be as simple as weight gain or mood changes to the more serious accusations of cancer and heart disease. Many doctors consider contraceptive pills to be responsible for depleting the body of vitamins.

Any woman considering taking the pill should be examined regularly for possible associated diseases. If you have a history of blood pressure, heart disease or phlebitis, or have a close relative who has any of these complaints, then you should look for another form of contraception.

● *Barrier contraception.*

Sheaths, caps (or diaphragms) and vaginal sponges are the oldest known form of contraception. Our ancestors used sheep's or pigs' intestines as sheaths, half-lemons as caps and sea sponges dipped in vinegar as vaginal sponges! These rely on mechanical rather than chemical elements to prevent the sperm from meeting the ovum. The modern versions of these are far superior in both quality and effectiveness when used correctly.

These contraceptive methods have a low user rate due to their poor aesthetic quality. Many couples find them distasteful to use and claim that they spoil the spontaneity of lovemaking. Although this is no doubt true, there is the advantage of avoiding any chemical change in the body, so being more 'natural'. In these days of high-risk sex, for people who are not faithful to one partner sheaths have the added benefit of preventing the spread of sexually transmitted diseases. Women who have used barrier methods are also unlikely to develop cancer of the cervix. The spermicides used in conjunction with barrier contraceptives are likewise useful in combating disease, but can occasionally produce unfortunate irritation of the delicate vaginal lining.

● *Intra-uterine devices (IUDs).*

These small devices are inserted through the cervix into the cavity of the womb. They are best suited to women who have already had a child. The reasons as to why they work are not completely clear, but it is thought that they prevent any new conceived foetus from implanting in the wall of the uterus. This means that theoretically it is possible each month to conceive and then abort a very early pregnancy. Many women find this thought distasteful and have moral objections.

There can be unpleasant side-effects to IUDs including heavy bleeding and some incidents of uterine infection. These pelvic infections can eventually lead to sterility, as the delicate fallopian tubes become scarred and eventually blocked. On the more positive side, IUDs do not interrupt the spontaneous flow of lovemaking, create no chemical changes in the body, and have a low failure rate, although not as low as the Pill.

● *'Natural contraception or rhythm method'.*
For those people who have moral, religious, medical or aesthetic objections to the above-mentioned contraceptive methods, there is an alternative which involves pinpointing the day of ovulation and avoiding sexual intercourse on that day plus one or two on either side. For this to be effective a woman has to be very much in touch with her ovulatory and menstrual rhythms. Ovulation usually occurs about 14 days after the first day of the prior menstrual period, although this can vary. Some women are aware of the precise day of ovulation as their natural vaginal secretions change in consistency, becoming less viscous and more copious. A chart plotting temperatures on each day will also indicate when ovulation has occurred.

A woman with irregular periods will have difficulty in using this method. It also requires a degree of self-discipline for couples to abstain from lovemaking on the days surrounding ovulation. As it is possible for sperm to live up to four days in the fallopian tubes, this method is obviously not the most reliable available.

MID-LIFE MALAISE

If you are over the age of 45, some of the observations made in this section may well sound a familiar note. Until recently the mid-life crisis was seen mainly as a 'woman's problem'. This is due to the obvious physical changes experienced in the menopause. Over the past 10 years it has become more widely accepted that the changes are also mental and emotional and affect both men and women. Emotional problems and depression, once accredited to hormonal disturbances associated with the menopausal phase, are part of a changing outlook on life. Many of the physical aches and pains are a result of a poor, unstable emotional state.

As you approach middle age you become aware that life is a finite journey. A period of 'confidence crisis' often follows.

Between the ages of 35 and 40 mortality becomes a reality, as do the obvious signs of ageing. This realisation may dawn slowly or strike suddenly. It can also bring about a feeling of being trapped with no way out except death. Every person must come to terms with this and deal with the accompanying repercussions in their own way.

Assessment of how one has performed in life and whether expectations have been achieved is common in mid-life. There are bound to have been disappointments along with the good times. Many people set themselves a target to have 'made it' by the time they reach 40; to have reached a certain position in their career or to have a certain material possession such as a particular type of house or car. As this sort of person approaches the late thirties, a desperate sense of 'needing to achieve' can set in, creating stress and preventing enjoyment of the present.

Many people feel concerned that they are becoming less attractive in the employment market, and worry about whether they will be able to get another job should they be made redundant. Worries about whether sex drive and personal attractiveness will diminish are also common in mid-life, as are fears of major health upsets. The figures show that the incidence of heart disease, cancer and other major illnesses increases during the forties. Keeping fit can become an uphill struggle, especially if health has been taken for granted up to now. It becomes more difficult to lose the extra pounds, and there is a definite slowing down with less energy to spare unless regular exercise is taken.

If your health has been put in jeopardy over the years through smoking, poor diet and little exercise, it is likely to falter and show signs of long-term damage in mid-life. The resulting mental turmoil often leads to depression. In a way, there is a sense of loss and a mourning period ensues. This can be associated with lost youth, dreams, expectations, even lost children as they become more independent and move away. These strains can rock even the seemingly steadiest of marriages, especially if communication has been poor. Women, and especially men, tend to test out their continuing attractiveness by engaging in extra-marital affairs.

Acceptance of the ageing process can bring about a real sense of peace. Although there is pain in allowing the dreams to vanish, once these have been let go, the pressure is relieved. However, this does not usually happen until the painful period of the crisis is over and the person has come to terms with his or her fears and ideas of what may happen as he or she approaches the second half of life. At the same time there will also be a realisation this this is not a rehearsal for life, there will be no action replays. Time which was there to be wasted is now seen as precious and to be used positively. This is possibly the basis for the phrase, 'life begins at 40.'

There are many positive aspects to be experienced in mid-life. The children are likely to be more independent, leaving you time to please yourselves more. Once a woman has reached the menopause there is more sexual freedom, as there is no longer the fear of becoming pregnant accidentally and no worries about having to use contraception. The rewards of climbing the career ladder are likely to be reaped in these middle years. And as a mature member of society your opinion is likely to be sought as you now have experience to share!

To get the most out of life after 40, attention to health is extremely important. Through attention to diet, regular exercise and having the right amounts of relaxation, you can operate as a confident, useful member of society with a lot to give and as much to gain from life. Because the cell renewal in your body is slower than in the past, it needs extra vitamins and the right foods to boost its defence systems. Vitamin E is especially useful for cell renewal. Take care to have your blood pressure checked every six months and always visit your doctor if you have any signs of ill-health such as abnormal bleeding, extreme lethargy, breathlessness, a prolonged cough or any unusual lump. Every two or three years a cervical smear should be taken from every woman who is, or has been sexually active, to test for abnormal cells. Many serious diseases can be cured in their early stages, so do not jeopardise your life because of fear. Remember, 50 per cent of octogenarians have been diagnosed as suffering from cancer at some time in their life!

SENIOR CITIZENS

Those lucky enough to have survived to old age deserve our respect and the opportunity to live out their days with dignity. Even when not in good health, the elderly person's experience of life and knowledge of what history has to tell us is of tremendous value to those who are younger. Even so, caring for an elderly or infirm relative puts a tremendous strain on any family. Because of the personal feelings involved it is not always advisable or practical to care for relations, but this does not mean that feelings of guilt are not harboured.

Many elderly people much prefer to stay in their own homes rather than enter an old people's home or live with their grown-up children. They want to keep a sense of independence and the ability to live their lives as they choose. The aged will outnumber the young in a decade or so. Large numbers usually dictate a certain amount of power, and one can only hope that increasing demand will lead to an improvement in services and support for the elderly. Retirement can be a peaceful, happy period of life if the person concerned has enough money to live a comfortable existence and the health to enjoy it. Although old age is the time of life when one has to cope with bereavement through loss of friends and spouse, most old people are quite resigned to facing their own death and have no fears. The few that are frightened lead uncomfortable and unhappy lives for their last few years.

Health problems in old age

There are a number of illnesses associated with old age which tend to be part of a generally failing body and particularly of brain failure. The problems associated with treatment mean that a failure in one system of the body may affect another, and so on in a domino fashion. Multiple conditions involving several body systems may cause the doctor to issue multiple prescriptions, with the risk of drug interaction and drug-induced disease. As the kidney and liver are often not functioning fully, the drugs cannot be detoxified and may slowly poison the whole system.

● *Chronic brain failure (dementia).*
This is due to the irreversible loss of brain cells. We are born with 10 million brain cells which die at a steady rate throughout our adult life. Dementia usually sets in when more than 50 per cent of these cells have been lost. This decline is obviously greater in people who have alcohol problems as alcohol destroys cells prematurely. The symptoms are loss of memory, impaired personality (a coarsening of character, which becomes more self-centred and less self-critical, with deteriorating standards), impairment of intellect and loss of dexterity. No active treatment exists for this sad condition and help must be mainly supportive. Treatment with drugs may only increase the confusion and upset balance.

● *Confusional states.*
Grave errors are sometimes made where dementia is diagnosed rather than a confusional state with a reversible cause. Inadequate circulation due to heart disease or anaemia may be a causative factor, as might a toxic reaction to drugs or confusion due to stress.

● *Falls, fits and faints.*
Thirty per cent of the elderly are afflicted by falls, usually from tripping over an object or from fainting. Epilepsy is rarer, as are drop attacks and impaired circulation to the cerebellum in the brain. Drop attacks are often associated with insufficient blood reaching the brain through the arteries in the neck.

● *Strokes.*
This is a major cause of death in the elderly, surpassed only by heart disease and cancer. Blood pressure is usually the most important precipitating factor. Strokes may be caused

by a blood clot in the brain or by a blood vessel bursting, causing a brain haemorrhage. Strokes classically produce loss of speech, paralysis of one side of the face and some of the opposite side of the body. There exists a particular minor type of stroke known as a transient ischaemic episode (TIE) where the blood supply is temporarily impaired and the patient has signs of a stroke but recovers fully.

- *Parkinson's disease.*

This is a disease of the brain which first causes tremor of the hands and can be a great source of embarrassment, especially when the teacup rattles in the saucer. Further symptoms may be drooling of saliva and problems associated with drinking, chewing and swallowing. The patient may shun company because he or she feels distressed by the symptoms. Drug treatment for Parkinson's disease is disappointing.

- *Psychiatric illness.*

The elderly constitute a psychologically vulnerable group and their psychiatric problems can distress both them and their relatives. Depression in the old is often associated with someone who when younger was obsessional, conscientious or introverted. In old age such depression is twice as common as dementia which it can mimic closely. Often only an antidepressant drug can distinguish the difference.

- *Hypothermia.*

Only 0.5 per cent of elderly people are hypothermic in cold weather. Ten per cent are borderline. The problem is caused by impairment to the body's heat regulation mechanism, evidenced by failure to shiver if cold or sweat when hot. The hypothermic patient is usually cold even in parts of the body which are usually warm, such as under the arms. The face becomes pale and puffy and the voice husky. If the body temperature falls below 32°C the patient becomes very lethargic, and below 27°C the patient will become comatose. Cold weather will worsen other conditions such as heart disease, bronchitis and influenza, which are a far worse risk to the health of an old person.

● *Rheumatism and arthritis.*

These chronic conditions affect most old people to a greater or lesser degree. The pain and stiffness experienced in the joints can be a cause of great suffering. Unfortunately, drugs often have unpleasant side-effects and do not ease the condition greatly. Regular exercise of the affected joints is of paramount importance. Diet should be low in fats, especially the saturated animal fats, and high in fresh fruits and vegetables. There are several herbal remedies such as alfalfa and nettle which can sometimes have a beneficial effect on rheumatism and arthritis.

Old people who live alone often lose the will to live and do not take care of themselves. They do not bother to make proper, nutritious meals for themselves and find it difficult to make new friends and improve their social life. The increasing number of old people's clubs at leisure centres encourage senior citizens to lead fuller, more active lives. Loneliness, a great worry for many people as they grow older, can be prevented if society includes the elderly as individuals with experience from which we can learn, rather than viewing them as a burden to be shunned.

6
The alternative first aid kit

Contents

Salt
Lemon
Honey
Ice (a bag of frozen peas will
    suffice)
Aloe vera plant
Tiger balm
Comfrey ointment
Alfalfa tablets
Garlic capsules
Olbas oil
Sage herbs
Sage and comfrey ointment
Paracetamol tables or syrup
    (sugar-free)
Mineral water
'Live' plain yoghurt
Cider apple vinegar
Ginger root capsules
Vinegar
Bicarbonate of soda
Sticking plasters
Bandages

For simple first aid it is quite unnecessary to have a home medicine cabinet full of sophisticated drugs and expensive proprietary remedies. Many of the items which you would find in any kitchen can be used medicinally in case of emergency. For instance, common salt may be used in a solution (½ teaspoon of salt to ¼ pint of warm boiled water) as a gargle for soothing sore throats, a mouthwash for mouth ulcers, or to clear the nasal passages in chronic sinusitis (see pages 124–5). The aloe vera plant can be kept for decorative purposes and doubles as a relief for burns and scalds. The sap contained in the stalks may be rubbed on the affected skin, soothing and helping to heal more quickly. A more detailed description follows of how these substances can be used for medicinal purposes.

Prevention and treatment of common ailments

Throughout this book we have stressed how important it is to care for and respect all aspects of your health so that you do not fall ill. However, even the healthiest people occasionally suffer irritating minor illnesses, especially following an emotional blow. If you are basically healthy you should be able to throw off most of these conditions within a few days. This chapter contains a few tips for treatment so that you will be incapacitated for the minimum time possible. If you continuously fall prey to current infections then your body is giving you a message to improve your standard of general health.

● *Bruising.*
Everyone, especially boisterous children, knock or bang themselves sometimes, resulting in cuts and bruises. However, if you regularly bruise perhaps you should consider the reason. For instance, are you trying to do everything in a rush or feeling so tired that you are more careless? If you appear to bruise easily you may be short of vitamin E, or your system may be slightly toxic and require cleansing.

Any hard blow to your body should immediately be treated locally with ice to prevent swelling and to lessen the bruising. (This is where the packet of frozen peas comes in handy!) If the injury is particularly severe, the affected part should be raised and the ice compressed on it. After about half an hour, the ice may be removed and comfrey ointment can be gently rubbed over the affected area. This should be repeated every few hours.

● *Burns.*
Should the burn be severe, a clean, cold cloth should be used to cover the affected area and the patient taken to the nearest hospital casualty department. Any minor burn or scald should be immediately immersed in cold water, not ice. If clothing is involved this should be removed as quickly as possible as it holds the heat on the skin, worsening the pain and the injury. Do not worry if skin peels away with the clothes as this will be dead anyway.

If the burn is minor, then the affected area may be kept immersed in cold water until the pain eases. The sap from an aloe vera plant can be spread over it, covering after with a clean cotton cloth. Ensure that this is not a fabric which will stick to the burn and peel away the healing skin.

● *Constipation.*
In 90 per cent of cases this is due to a sluggish system caused by poor diet and lack of dietary fibre. Habitual and long-term constipation can eventually lead to chronic bowel problems such as piles, diverticulitis and, in some cases, cancer. Lack of vitamins B complex and B1 may be an additional 'cause in some cases.

Obviously, the first line of action should be to increase the intake of fibre with inclusion in the diet of fresh fruit, vegetables and wholegrain products such as wholemeal bread and brown rice. Instead of coffee and tea, fruit juices and copious amounts of mineral water should be consumed. Brisk exercise such as walking, cycling or jogging will help to stir up a sluggish system.

Keep the use of purgatives to the very minimum. These will have the effect of making the natural bowel movements become more lazy in the long run.

● *Coughs and colds.*
Some naturopaths consider that the common cold is a way the body has of reacting to an imbalance in the system and cleansing impurities which have built up. The medical profession sees it purely as a viral infection. The truth probably lies somewhere between these two extremes. Often a cold will strike when you are at a low ebb emotionally or physically. A good preventive measure is the regular taking of garlic capsules. (Buy the sort which have no aftertaste so that you keep your friends!) Garlic is a 'natural antibiotic' and aids the cleansing of the whole system. Vitamins, especially vitamin C, are important because they help to build our immunity to germs.

Proprietary cold remedies are expensive and not much use. If you feel as though you are starting a cold and have an itchy, sore throat try gargling with warm salt water each hour. This can often keep the cold from developing any further. Drink copious amounts of fluids. Hot lemon and honey infusions are especially useful as they contain antiseptic properties. Simple paracetamol tablets will help to relieve any accompanying aches and pains. Continue taking the garlic capsules. Antibiotics are of no use at this stage because colds are viral rather than bacterial in origin. For your blocked nose, smear a little olbas oil under your nostrils and sprinkle some on your pillow to help you breathe during the night. Karvol capsules broken on to a handkerchief and inhaled have the same effect.

One misery of a cold is the bright red, sore nose from continual use of a handkerchief. Sage and comfrey ointment is marvellous for reducing the inflammation. If your cold starts to dry up leaving your sinuses blocked with thickened mucus, you may alleviate it by inhalation of the steam from friars balsam in boiling water. Follow this with a weak, warm salt solution to clear the nasal passages. You may do this by sniffing the water up your nose, tilting back your head and bringing the fluid into your mouth where you can spit it out. This is best done in private as it is a rather revolting, though very useful, process! Reduce the amount of alcohol you consume as this has the effect of drying out the sinuses, leading to pain which is often excruciating. All dairy products, especially milk, should be strictly limited, as should sugary substances as these produce excess mucus.

Coughing is an important reflex to protect the delicate bronchial tubes and their linings. If you have a persistent cough you should have your chest examined by a doctor to ensure that the cough does not have a serious cause. Most coughs develop as a result of a cold. Mucus drips down the back of the throat, irritating the cough reflex. Some productive coughs are due to a chest infection which is best treated with antibiotics under medical supervision. Garlic capsules, once again, will help to relieve a cough following a cold.

● *Cystitis.*
This unfortunate condition is mainly confined to women. This is due to the fact that women have a short, straight passage leading out from the bladder whereas men have a longer, more convoluted one. This means that in women bacteria find their way more easily into the bladder, causing symptoms associated with inflammation.

Passing of urine is frequent, painful and sometimes contains blood. This may be accompanied by low stomach pain and a raised temperature. The pain when passing urine is caused by high acidity, and this should be diluted by drinking copious amounts of fluids. Antibiotics are often necessary to get rid of the infection. Remember the whole course must be finished to prevent recurrence.

If you are prone to cystitis then investigation may be necessary to discount involvement of the kidneys. Very often irritation of the urethra during sexual intercourse is a cause of cystitis. Women should pass water before and after (especially after) intercourse to flush out the urethra. Hygiene is obviously important, but take care not to use harsh soaps in the delicate vulval area as these may irritate the skin and reduce immunity to infection.

- *Diarrhoea*.

This unpleasant condition is mainly infective in origin, although it is sometimes caused by leakage past the motions contained in the bowels of severely constipated people. It may also be instigated by the 'fight or flight' reflex when you are nervous or frightened.

Your body is doing its level best to rid your system of something which may cause it harm. Allow it to do this rather than stop the diarrhoea with drugs. Rest your digestive system for at least 12 hours, taking only occasional small sips of mineral water. (We have found the naturally fizzy spa water best for this purpose.) Natural 'live' yoghurt should then be taken, two tablespoons every hour for the next 12 hours. This contains bacteria which help to fortify the defences contained in your bowels. Warm apple cider vinegar and honey may be drunk along with the mineral water. Think of this as a cleansing exercise. After 24 hours you may start to eat small regular amounts of food such as wholemeal bread, brown rice or bananas. Aim to keep off milk and sugary products for at least another 24 hours. *Never* take an antibiotic if you have diarrhoea as this will worsen the condition and prolong your suffering.

- *Headaches*.

Persistent headaches are very worrying for the sufferer. They are most commonly caused by stress but can be brought on by eye strain, allergy to food substances or sinusitis. There are more serious causes, and you should visit your general practitioner for investigation if you suffer from persistent headaches.

Migraine is frequently associated with diarrhoea, vomiting and dizziness. The pain is generally confined to one side of the head. Anxiety usually plays a large part in the onset of migraine, but it may also be caused by certain substances such as red wine, chocolate and avocado pears. Self-hypnosis is extremely effective in combating migraine, and the herbal remedy feverfew has also been shown to be helpful.

For a severe tension headache, painkillers are often useless. Relaxation is the key to relieving the contracted muscles of the scalp and neck which cause the headache. Worry about the headache often leads to worsening of the condition. Anxiety is a totally destructive part of modern life, and is at the root of many modern diseases. Worrying about the future, or about people close to you, can become a very bad habit. Often worry is (mis)taken as a sign that a person cares for another, but it can be bound up with feelings of guilt. Once these feelings have been examined and separated, then worry can be abandoned. The energy used up in worrying can be channelled constructively to improve situations you dislike. Remember, most things you worry about never actually happen!

● *Mouth ulcers.*
These irritating eruptions may be due to lack of vitamins A or C, or to poor oral hygiene. Use of badly washed cutlery might also be responsible.

Rinsing the mouth with salt water is quite as effective as the use of proprietary brands of mouthwash. An infusion of sage or comfrey herbs used as a mouthwash will also help to reduce the swelling. Regular outbreaks of mouth ulcers should be checked by your doctor to exclude any underlying cause.

● *Muscular aches and pains.*
These may be due to rheumatism and fibrositis, or may be the result of strenuous exercise, nervous tension or poor posture. Generally speaking muscles like warmth, and the application of a heat lamp or hot water bottle locally is often of great benefit. Paradoxically, the application of ice is also useful as this will bring about a 'rebound' action where the blood will rush to the affected part once the ice is removed. Ointments such as tiger balm, which make the skin feel warm when rubbed on, are also comforting. Perhaps best of all is a good massage of the affected muscle group by expert or loving hands!

● *Sore throats.*
Inflammation of the throat is usually due to infection or

irritation by fumes or toxic substances. Alcohol, especially neat spirits, dries out the delicate throat membranes, creating or worsening soreness, and should be avoided when you have a throat infection. Constriction of the throat during nervous tension depletes the blood supply resulting in a sore throat.

Sage tea may be drunk regularly to reduce the inflammation and garlic capsules taken if there is some infection present. If you suffer from a chronic sore throat, give up drinking alcohol and eating spicy food for a period of a month to six weeks in order to allow the membranes to heal.

● *Thrush*.

This is a fungal infection in women which affects the vaginal membranes and may be passed via sexual contact to male partners. Unfortunately, the spores can be harboured by men without inducing symptoms so that the female sexual partners become reinfected. New-born babies often become infected in their mouths as they are passing through the birth canal.

In women the symptoms are itching, soreness, and a heavy yellow-green discharge from the vagina. A white, speckled rash is apparent (hence' the name 'thrush') inside the vagina which if rubbed leaves raw patches which bleed. All very unpleasant.

As this is a fungal infection it thrives in warm, damp conditions and tends to recur once it has found a home. Certain imbalances in the body enable it to recur. Antibiotics are a prime cause of body imbalances and this is as good a reason as any for avoiding them whenever possible. Many women find they have thrush throughout their pregnancies. Alcohol, sugar and yeast products in the diet also encourage its reappearance. When you are trying to rid yourself of this nuisance, keep away from these substances throughout your treatment.

Natural 'live' yoghurt contains the bacteria which will fight the fungal infection. Include this in your diet for a week, and in the same period choose two or three consecutive nights when you immerse a tampon into yoghurt until the yoghurt is absorbed and then insert the tampon high into the vagina. Often the best time for this is the few days following your period, a time when many women find thrush has returned. If you have a steady sexual partner he should apply the yoghurt as an ointment around the penis, particularly under his foreskin. Ensure that you and your partner carry out the treatment simultaneously to avoid reinfection.

● *Vomiting.*
As with diarrhoea, vomiting is usually the result of infection through bad food. It may also be a reaction to an irritating substance such as alcohol, a direct result of overeating, or be due to anxiety or motion sickness.

Food poisoning will produce symptoms of dizziness, sweating and diarrhoea accompanied by vomiting within a few hours of eating the infected food. In some cases this can be very serious, especially in the very young or the elderly. Treatment should be medically supervised to avoid the danger of dehydration occurring.

Should you start vomiting, allow your stomach to rest for at least 12 hours. Even sips of water can restart the vomiting reflex. Once you are feeling more settled, take three garlic capsules and a spoonful of 'live' yoghurt. During the next 12 hours drink only mineral water (the natural fizzy type is best in this case). Repeat the garlic capsules, two every four hours over the next 24 hours. Remember that your system has now been cleansed and build your eating pattern appropriately by starting with some brown rice and a little fruit. Avoid dairy products, sugar and very salty or fried food for a few days. Stay off spicy food and alcohol over the next week.

If you know that you suffer from motion sickness, ensure that you do not eat for at least an hour before you begin your journey and sit in the front of the vehicle if possible. Ginger root capsules may help to prevent vomiting and are quite safe to give to children.

● *Depression.*
Depressive illness is a very common, though certainly not

simple, condition. It can range from feeling 'under the weather' or 'a bit down' to a seriously debilitating psychotic illness requiring hospital treatment. The reasons for the onset of depression are many and range from simple vitamin deficiency to mourning the loss of a loved one.

Recognising depressive illness is not always easy, particularly if there is a slow decline and no obvious causes. Some patients are capable of appearing cheerful and it is not at all easy to spot the 'smiling depressive'. Clues may be found in lack of care for appearance or sudden loss of weight. Lethargy and lack of interest are common signs of depression. A patient may find it difficult to sleep, or may wake very early in the morning with all manner of worries but find it difficult to raise him- or herself from bed. Phobic behaviour may develop, such as agoraphobia, or alternatively obsessive behaviour, for instance where the patient checks and rechecks whether he or she has switched all the lights off before going to bed. Above all the patient feels guilty for being ill and burdensome to close relatives.

Depression is part of the mourning process. Loss, whether it is of a beloved person, job or home, produces feelings which follow a certain pattern. There is initial disbelief, followed by denial then anger. Depression is the next stage and finally acceptance. If any of these stages are missed then depression is likely to be lasting until worked through. Anger is the most commonly excluded stage because of the guilt which people feel about anger. If a recently bereaved person eulogises the dead relative or friend, this is a danger signal warning that the person is unable to face the anger he or she feels at being left alone, and the mourning process becomes 'stuck'. Mourning is a part of life and we mourn the passing of stages throughout life. Frequently, internalised anger is at the root of depression. Lengthy counselling or psychotherapy may be required to free the submerged emotions and help the patient come to terms with feelings.

In some cases, depression can ultimately be very positive. For example, if you become depressed but learn what lies at the root of your illness, this can be a springboard to making changes for the better. People who have successfully come through a depressive illness frequently have a greater insight into their own personality and are stronger for their experience. Unfortunately, a minority of those who fall into deep depression find it impossible to continue their lives and attempt to commit suicide. These are the cases which are admitted to hospital for their own safety.

The complexity of the human psyche precludes the use of one straightforward approach towards depressive patients. Each person's illness is as individual as he or she is. Drug treatment is precarious and often has unpleasant side-effects. The depression is also likely to recur if its origins have not been examined. There is an unfortunate trend in psychiatry towards drug therapy which does not take into account the uniqueness of every patient which is an integral factor in their illness. This attitude among many psychiatrists leads to a trial-and-error management of patients, where different drugs are tested over a period of time until the 'right' one is found. We can only hope that this fashion may be overturned with the next generation of doctors.

Suggested further reading

Allergies — What Everyone Should Know, Keith Mumby (London, Unwin Paperbacks)

Birth Reborn, Michael Odent (London, Souvenir Press)

Menopause — The Best Years of Your Life, Ada Khan and Linda Hughey Holt (London, Bloomsbury)

Nutrition against Disease, Roger Williams (London, Pitman)

Stretch and Relax, Maxine Tobias and Mary Stewart (Dorling Kindersley)

The Joy Of Stress, J. Hanson (London, Pan Books)

The New Cook Book, Miriam Polunin (London, Macdonald)

Who's Having Your Baby? Beverley Lawrence Beech (Camden Press)

Useful addresses

The Food Allergy Association
9 Mill Lane
Shoreham-by-Sea
West Sussex

Institute of Complementary
  Medicine
21 Portland Place
London W1N 3AF